The first in a remarkable series

THE ULTIMATE PUBLISHING HOUSE (TUPH)
US HEADQUARTERS
The Ultimate Publishing House (TUPH)
P.O. Box 1204, Cypress, Texas, U.S.A. 77410

49540 – 80 Glen Shields Avenue, Toronto, Ontario, Canada L4K 2B0

Telephone: 647-883-1758 Fax: 416-228-2598

www.ultimatepublishinghouse.com and www.tbookseries.com
E-mail: info@ultimatepublishinghouse.com

US OFFICE: Ordering Information
Quantity Sales: COMPANIES, ORGANIZATIONS, INSTITUTIONS, AND INDUSTRY PUBLICATIONS.

Quantity discounts are available on bulk purchases of this book for reselling, educational purposes, subscription incentives, gifts, sponsorship, or fundraising. Unique books or book excerpts can also be fashioned to suit specific needs such as private labeling with your logo on the cover and a message from or a message printed on the second page of the book. For more information, please contact our Special Sales Department at The Ultimate Publishing House. Orders for college textbook or course adoption use.

Please contact The Ultimate Publishing House Tel: 647-883-1758
TUPH is a registered trademark of The Ultimate Publishing House

Contributing Cover Design by Bridget Braun
Inside Page Layout by Bridget Braun

Printed in the United States.

North America's Top Doctors, by Felicia Pizzonia, R.H.N.
ISBN: 978-0-9819398-9-6

t SERIES

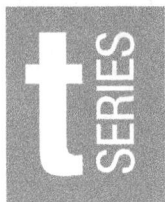

NORTH AMERICA'S **TOP DOCTORS**

SHARE SECRETS TO ANTI-AGING & WELLNESS

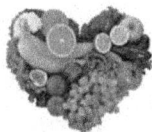

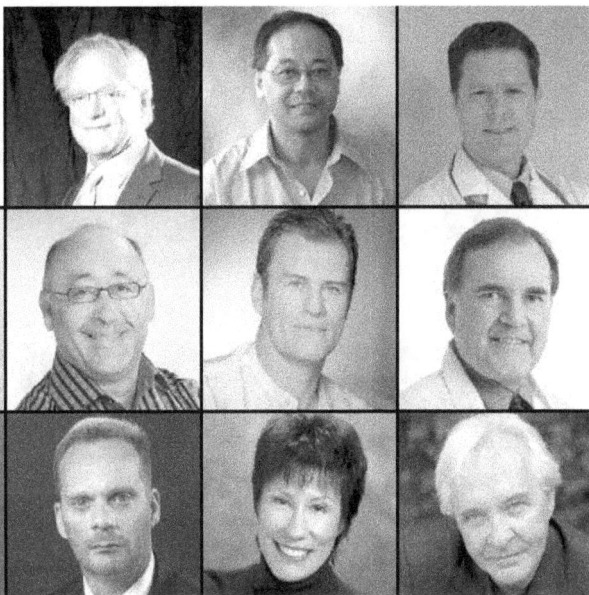

FEATURING: Dr. Tom Barnard • Dr. Larry Chan • Dr. Screven Edgerton

Dr. David Garcia • Dr. Roger Garcia • Dr. Bruce Hoffman • Dr. Randy LaFrom

Dr. Susan Linder • Dr. Paul Savage • Dr. Pamela Smith • Dr. Andrew Wojcicki

FIRST EDITION

DISCLAIMER

North America's Top Doctors is not intended to diagnose or prescribe any treatment for any medical or psychological condition(s), nor are there any claims or offers to prevent, diagnose, treat, mitigate, or cure any medical or psychological conditions.

The authors and publisher specifically disclaim all responsibility for any liability, loss, or risk, personal or otherwise, that is incurred as a consequence (directly or indirectly) of any inaccurate information of the chapters and interviews of this book.

The book contains the ideas and opinions of its authors and is intended solely to provide helpful information. It is offered with the understanding that the authors and publisher are not engaged in rendering medical, health, or any other kind of personal/professional services in the book.

The reader should consult his or her medical, health, or other competent professional before adopting any of the suggestions in the book.

The authors and publisher specifically disclaim all responsibility for any liability, loss, or risk, personal or otherwise, that is incurred as a consequence (directly or indirectly) of the use and application of any of the contents of this book. The book contains the following disclaimer:

The names of people mentioned in the case studies published within the book have been changed to protect the people's identity.

DISCLAIMER

ACKNOWLEDGMENTS

There are many people apart from the authors who are involved in creating a book - from the time it's first conceived to the time it becomes a printed bestseller. As a collective, we would like to acknowledge their many contributions.

First of all, we would like to thank Felicia Pizzonia of The Ultimate Publishing House, without whom none of this would have been possible. It was her thoughtful interviewing style and intense interest in the topics of anti-aging and wellness that led to the birth of this book. Her attention to detail and dedication as she worked with us to edit each chapter - making it thorough, complete, and most of all, accurate - is very much appreciated. We thank her immensely.

Secondly, we are indebted to our teachers, institutions, and professional colleagues who have informed and supported us throughout our careers. Many still provide advice, guidance, and collaboration as we learn and practice with patients day-to-day. They've shared their own case studies and experiences with us. They've also helped care for our patients as we travel to conferences to further our professional studies in each of our specialties. Thank you for all your efforts to support us in this way.

Thirdly, we would like to express our gratitude to our families and loved ones, who, over the years, have given us time, patience and support as we trained, practiced, and developed our skills as doctors. They are too numerous to mention here individually. We've spent so many hours away from them to do our jobs as doctors. What we do can be stressful and difficult at times, but without their love and support, it would be even more so. We are forever grateful for you.

And last but not least, we'd like to thank our patients. You are what we live for. You allow us to care for you, you teach us, and you share your most personal information with us. You trust us by putting your lives in our hands, and that's a privilege with which we take the utmost care. We grow as you heal and rejoice in your recovery from illness. As anti-aging specialists, we take a special pride in helping to maintain your quality of life as you get older and face new health challenges. Thank you for placing your health in our trust.

We remain forever in your debt and in your service. We hope this book will become a valuable tool and reference in helping you to stay healthy throughout your entire life.

All the best,

Dr. Thomas Barnard, Dr. Larry Chan, Dr. Screven Edgerton, Dr. David Garcia, Dr. Roger Garcia, Dr. Bruce Hoffman, Dr. Randall LaFrom, Dr. Susan Linder, Dr. Paul Savage, Dr. Pamela Smith, and Dr. Andrew Wojcicki

SECOND EDITION COMING OUT 2012!

DEDICATION

My wish is for all of the people of the world to read this book and benefit from the information provided by some of the world's greatest doctors. Living a life of good quality health is the key to achieving success in all aspects of life. This book is the key to smoothing the progress toward obtaining health, longevity, and success. Life is meant to be joyful; take care of yourself, your family, and friends.

Wishing all of you good health and vitality.

With love,

Felicia Pizzonia

TABLE OF CONTENTS

INTRODUCTION

The greatest wealth is health. ~ *Virgil*

The power of love to change bodies is legendary, built into folklore, common sense, and everyday experience. Love moves the flesh, it pushes matter around... Throughout history, "tender loving care" has uniformly been recognized as a valuable element in healing. ~ *Larry Dossey*

We all want to live long and gracefully. Since I was fifteen years old, I was immersed in and passionate about health and nutrition. I was blessed as a book publisher and partner of The Ultimate Publishing House to meet incredible doctor-authors. I learned so much about health and anti-aging that I felt the need to create a book that offered amazing information to help people find the way to good health. I decided to write a book and interview the top doctors in North America's anti-aging field. What better way to learn about health than to learn from the best in North America?

Most of us, when we hear the term "anti-aging," think of removing wrinkles and improving our body image, but that is only the outside packaging. True anti-aging means building health for a longer life and staving off degenerative diseases that make life miserable and ultimately shorten our lives. Who wants to live to a hundred with perfect skin and a slim body if it means suffering with osteoporosis, having activities limited by heart disease or emphysema, or dealing with the side effects of cancer treatment? Real anti-aging involves building good health to maintain strength and energy so that we can enjoy our later years and truly live life to the fullest. The result will include the health of our skin as it naturally reflects our inner glow. Prevention is the key to good health. This includes daily exercise, good sleep, healthy nutrition, good supplementation of vitamins and minerals, energy healing, and good quality alkaline water.

Anti-aging is also a matter of attitude. Attitude sets the stage for your life's journey and health. You are here to experience joy.

Enjoy reading the book and check out www.tbookseries.com. To connect with the doctors in the book, e-mail us at doctors@tbookseries.com.

Don't forget to check back for the second edition of North America's Top Doctors coming out in 2012.

To your health,

Felicia Pizzonia, R.H.N.
Ultimate Publishing House, Partner
Health Activist and Nutrition Dealer

www.ultimatepublishinghouse.com
www.medimarketingarm.com

CHAPTER ONE

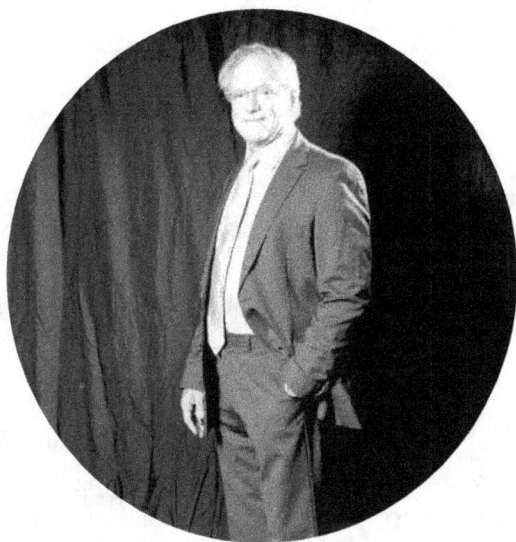

Dr. Thomas Barnard:

Insulin Resistance and Diabetes

CHAPTER ONE

Dr. Thomas Barnard:
Insulin Resistance and Diabetes

There is a crisis today: an epidemic rise in the number of people with diabetes, insulin resistance, and obesity. The Chinese have an interesting way of looking at a crisis. When you look at the word "crisis" in Chinese, it contains characters both for danger and for opportunity.

The danger is obvious. I see young children coming into my practice, and they are already straining their pancreas, forcing it to put out large amounts of insulin to try to keep their blood sugar normal after a meal.

And as we age, one characteristic that develops is a difficulty with insulin and glucose interaction. That, of course, contributes to one of the other aging hallmarks, inflammation, and to a decline in our ability to effectively produce energy. This process is starting around the world at a younger and younger age. So, it's imperative that we recognize how significant this issue is and reverse it.

That's where the opportunity comes in. As doctors, we can look at your metabolism today and get an idea of where you're going in the future. It's like Mark Twain said: If you don't change directions, you'll wind up where you're heading. We take the metabolic direction a person is heading and correct it if it's not optimal. We have the ability to look at a person's unique physiology and biochemical challenges and create a program just for them.

It's exciting for me as a physician to be working in this day and age. With every patient I see — whatever age, whatever the concerns — I have the ability to measure their insulin resistance, — as well as every vitamin, mineral, and amino acid in their bodies — and correct what's missing. I can have such an impact on a person's immediate energy levels and their enjoyment of everyday life.

For example, my mother-in-law, a woman in her late seventies, was in my office not too long ago. She had been complaining for years of joint pain and fatigue. Through an analysis, I found out that she was not only insulin resistant, but had a number of nutritional deficits and some hormonal issues to balance. Once I fixed those deficits, her quality of life improved dramatically.

What is insulin, and how does it play a role in diabetes? Anybody watching TV or reading the newspaper has no doubt heard the terms. Our bodies are marvelously complex machines. They bring in energy and process that energy into fuel that powers our body and all its functions. Insulin, a hormone secreted by the pancreas, allows the fuel derived from carbohydrates and proteins in our diets to be burned in the furnaces in every cell in the body.

The pancreas responds in an intricate and coordinated way to the amount of food we take in and releases the right amount of insulin to keep the level of sugar in our blood consistent. We can, over time, lose the ability to produce insulin. But more commonly, what happens is that we produce insulin, but when it gets to cells in the body – the heart, lungs, muscle, or brain – those cells become resistant. The cells resist the ability of insulin to allow the fuel (glucose, for example) to enter the cell to be burned for energy.

The way insulin works is that it has to come into contact with a cell's membrane, a selective barrier that surrounds the cell. Insulin is then recognized by a port in the barrier, bound to the molecule and allowed to enter the cell. Then, insulin has to open up a gate that allows sugar to be absorbed and taken by a transport molecule inside the cell to go into the "furnace" and make heat for daily living.

Resistance to insulin occurs for lots of reasons. Sometimes, that receptor may not have the right building blocks to allow insulin to be recognized easily. It may then take higher and higher levels of insulin to push open that gate that insulin controls. That's when we develop resistance to the effects of insulin.

Rather than taking just a little bit of insulin to maintain a normal, relatively low blood sugar (glucose) level throughout the day, we require increasingly higher levels of insulin, especially after eating a meal, to keep blood sugar normal.

At first, we have a blood sugar rise after a meal. Then, we get a whole lot of insulin that's produced because we're relatively resistant to its effects. Eventually, there's so much insulin produced and it pushes so hard on the cell membranes that the blood sugar falls very quickly. The low blood sugar can be developed a few hours after a meal, so there's a seesaw effect. And that's difficult for your quality of life.

In diabetes prevention trials in the United States, United Kingdom, and Finland, all of them showed that the best way to correct insulin resistance is through diet and lifestyle. So that's the foundation of everything we do in our practice. In our approach, we have the ability to not only use diet and lifestyle approaches, but to tailor them to a person's own physiology and make the approaches so much more effective.

Lifestyle is our foundation, but we can also amplify the impact of lifestyle by truly understanding an individual's nutritional requirements and help a person reverse insulin resistance. We can also help a person reverse the changes that occur in body composition as they age. When we age, we tend to gain fat, especially around the middle of the body. Fat is an insulin-resistant tissue. As we continue to gain fat, we fill up the fat cells to the point where they become "overfull," and then fat deposits in many other places as well, like the liver, muscle, and bone marrow. This is a marker of the "overconsumptive undernutrition" so much a part of our current lifestyle and diet. It is both the cause of, and the result of, the accumulation of insulin-resistant body mass.

As well, as we age, we tend to lose bone and muscle, the lean body mass that's insulin sensitive. Reversing insulin resistance helps us maintain lean body mass, reduce fat, and maintain insulin sensitivity. Insulin sensitivity is both the cause of, and the result of, a healthy body composition. When we maintain a healthy balance of lean and fat mass, the insulin that our pancreas secretes in response to foods and metabolic demands is used efficiently, a little insulin goes a long way, and we can control our physiology with minimal insulin effort, thus avoiding the negative impact of high insulin levels in terms of accumulation of excess fat and concomitant excess inflammation.

As noted, one of the hallmarks of high insulin levels is the depositing of fat around the organs of the abdomen and in the organs themselves. A good example is fat in the liver. Accumulated fat in the liver has become the leading reason why people in North America have liver failure – even more than the viral infection hepatitis or alcoholism. It's astonishingly prevalent and something we really have to guard against.

These days, our society has readily available fast food, which allows people to take in calories greatly in excess of their insulin hormone's ability to drive those calories into the muscle to be burned as fuel. As a result, this extra energy gets deposited as fat.

We as a society also have spent a lot of time blaming the victim: you eat too much, you don't exercise enough, you sit in front of the TV, you get fat. All of those things will eventually make you become diabetic.

That's been the historical way of thinking.

But in the last few years, what's become clear is that the whole process is accelerated greatly by exposure to environmental pollutants. Some people can be fat, but when that fat is biopsied and there are no pollutants in it, they don't tend to become diabetic. The insulin resistance of the same overweight person who's been exposed to organic pollutants, organophosphates, and organocholorines (all of which accumulate in the fat) is higher for reasons that aren't entirely clear. It's been seen in soldiers who were exposed to Agent Orange and in farm workers exposed to pesticides.

These organic pollutants tend to magnify themselves in foods highest up the food chain. For example, it's been discovered that the most contaminated breast milk in the world comes from Inuit women on Baffin Island in the Canadian Arctic, a relatively isolated and pristine place. Organic pollutants are precipitated into the cold Arctic Ocean, first getting into the plankton, then small fish, and bigger fish and eventually, into sea mammals such as seals that are the basis of the Inuit diet. These people are eating very high on the food chain, and the pollutants that lead to diabetes are magnified in their diets.

The same applies to us. If we eat a diet of animals that have eaten plants grown with pesticides, the animal has these chemicals concentrated in its body and in its fat. When we eat the animal, we absorb the fat and chemicals, too.

Over the years, we've also been taught myths about dieting. Some years ago, the argument was made that if a person is getting fat and has high cholesterol, it must come from fat in his or her diet. So by eating a low-fat diet, you would reduce your risk of heart disease. Food manufacturers believed that and created diets that were low in fat, but they replaced that fat with sugar.

Over the last couple of decades, our children have been exposed to diets that are high in processed simple carbohydrates. These carbs are sugars that create stress on the body's insulin and glucose machinery. It's as if you are doing a glucose challenge every day when you drink a can of soda, which has the equivalent of ten to fifteen teaspoons of sugar in every can. And some people drink several cans a day!

Even worse, we took out sugar and replaced it with high fructose corn syrup, which our bodies handle even more poorly and seem to generate insulin resistance directly. And, artificial sweeteners, with the exception of a few natural ones like stevia (a plant extract), are not helping. They have not been shown to help people lose weight and even have their own toxicities.

Our insulin resistance stems from these issues: we cut out fat and replaced it with sugar, we consume more calories and are less active than we used to be, and there are more environmental contaminants. It's no good arguing over the type of diet – high protein, carbs, no carbs – that you should follow. What you should do is find a diet of foods that you love, select unprocessed foods that are part of your cultural heritage, moderate your portion size, and choose fruits and vegetables that are high in the protective colorful phytochemicals.

Whatever it is, you want to choose a kind of diet that you can successfully maintain.

Choose high quality foods. Don't drink soda. Drink plenty of water. Take carbohydrates in their natural, unprocessed form, such as beans, legumes, or oatmeal. Use animal products in moderation. Stay away from foods with too much saturated fat and even less contaminated saturated fat. If you're going to eat beef, eat beef from cows that were raised as cows have always been, eating grass instead of grain.

Eat high-quality proteins such as fish. Remember that even plants themselves have plenty of protein. Rice, for example, is 11 percent protein. Among plants, the real protein winners are legumes and beans.

Make sure the plants you're eating are not hybridized or genetically modified species. And when possible, eat locally grown foods that aren't years away from the field and still contain some good nutrition. Don't eat foods out of a box or from the freezer.

Eat fresh fruits and vegetables in season. We used to believe that the cancer or heart disease-reducing properties of plants were primarily because of their high vitamin and mineral content. We now know that in addition to vitamins and minerals, plants provide colorful phytochemicals. Diets rich in vegetables, fruit, and whole grains protect us from high insulin levels, because we absorb sugars more slowly when they're in the presence of these phytochemicals, especially in the setting of the inherent high-fiber content of the vegetable or fruit. And the phytochemicals are also powerful anti-oxidant protection in their own right, protecting vulnerable tissues like the retina of the eye and the energy centers of every cell, the mitochondria, which depend on the powerful protective ability of the phytochemicals in our diet for protection from the oxidative stresses inherent in their job of energy creation in each cell. Vive le phytochemicals!

You also want to choose fats that are anti-inflammatory. Foods that contain the anti-inflammatory omega-3 fatty acids include salmon and other fish, flax, hemp, or algae. The source of the food is important. Farmed fish like tilapia doesn't have much omega-3 – and little anti-inflammatory effect – in it at all. And depending on what the farmed fish is fed, it can be contaminated with its own pesticides and residue.

Make sensible choices, and try not to get stuck in a yo-yo pattern of weight gain and loss. Ideally, you should have a relatively small percentage of body fat, or at least one that's not excessive and relatively consistent. Aim to maintain an exercise pattern of walking, running, or resistance training mixed with cardio training of about an hour a day. If you do some sort of physical activity right up until the end of your life, that gives you the best chance of avoiding insulin resistance and diabetes.

People don't need to eat huge amounts of calories with the exception of when they're young and growing, pregnant or breastfeeding, or working out very hard. If you choose foods of a high quality that go along with your personal tastes and control portions, you'll do very well.

The majority of people with diabetes in our society have type 2, where they're making plenty of insulin but have developed insulin resistance. We can correct that by making their receptors rich in omega-3 fats. Vitamin D is also important, and its levels should be kept at the upper end of normal. Chromium is also needed, because the mineral is absent in the soil. Coenzyme Q10 and alpha-lipoic acid and acetyl-L-carnitine are also key in energy production. Diabetics also need magnesium, potassium, B vitamins, folic acid (found in leafy green 'foliage' vegetables), lycopene (found in tomatoes, watermelon, and strawberries), resveratrol (found in red wine and red grapes), and zinc.

There's another major issue of aging that's tied to insulin resistance and diabetes. If you live to be eighty years old in Canada or the United States, there's a 50 percent chance you will develop dementia or Alzheimer's disease. Some are calling Alzheimer's disease or age-related memory loss type 3 diabetes, and that makes the topics of insulin resistance and diabetes that much more important to address in our aging process.

All of us would love to be a hundred, a hundred and ten years old with our families, partners, children, or ourselves, as long as we are capable and active people. That's possible by maintaining an active lifestyle and making the right kind of choices and with colorful fruits and vegetables in your diet. When choosing any food, look at it and ask the following question: Is this the best food for my body, at this time in my life, and will it improve my level of activity, my level of health? Will it improve how I feel, or will it have a negative impact?

If you ask those questions, you're making a conscious choice to take good care of yourself and make your long life a healthy one.

Dr. Thomas Barnard

Dr. Thomas Barnard has been a pioneer in the field of nutritional medicine and health since 1988. He's an internationally known speaker as well as a radio and TV personality in anti-aging and regenerative medicine. He's the medical director of Fresh Medical Spa in Windsor, Ontario, where he practices aesthetic medical techniques, including non-invasive body sculpting, facial rejuvenation, Botox, bioidentical hormone balancing, and weight-loss programs.

Dr. Barnard is a graduate of Cornell University and University of Rochester School of Medicine, and he performed his residency in family and emergency medicine at Rutgers University Medical School. He's board certified in family practice, laser medicine, and emergency medicine and has a fellowship in anti-aging, functional, and regenerative medicine. He has also taught at the University of Western Ontario, the University of Guelph, and the University of South Florida.

Dr. Barnard is the author of *Defeating Diabetes* (2003), which emphasizes the power of whole-foods diets in reversing the epidemic of type 2 diabetes. He's currently working on his Master of Science degree in Medicine with a concentration in metabolism and nutrition at the University of South Florida Medical School.

Dr. Thomas Barnard
Fresh Medical Spa
2430 Dougall Avenue
Windsor, Ontario, Canada
N8X 1T2

Phone: 519-9267-8400
E-mail: freshmedicalspa@mdirect.net
www.freshmedicalspa.com

CHAPTER TWO

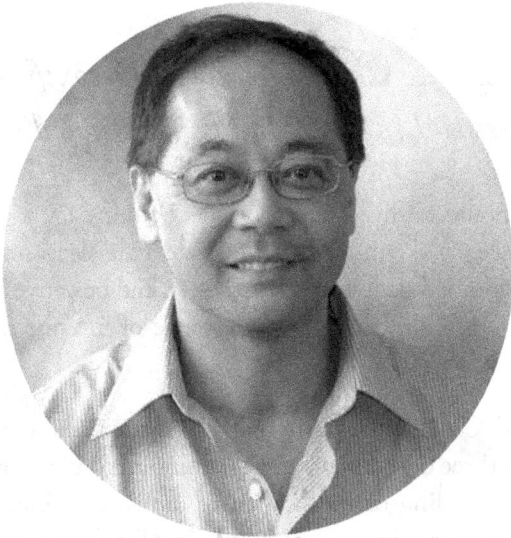

Dr. Lawrence Chan:

Metabolic Detoxification –
Essential in Age Management Medicine

CHAPTER TWO

Dr. Lawrence Chan: Metabolic Detoxification – Essential in Age Management Medicine

L ife should be lived simply. One shouldn't try to make it too complex: wake up, exercise, get adequate sleep/rest, be around like-minded people and loved ones, and be active and engaged in the larger community. That's the essence of life one should try to embrace.

I've practiced Chinese and Alternative medicine as a Naturopathic Physician for three decades and engage this philosophy as a foundation for my understanding of the human condition and how we interact with the environment in order to maintain a life filled with health and vitality.

Consider the unifying philosophy of the "Triad of Health" as it applies to the human condition:

1. Structural (musculoskeletal)
2. Bio-chemical (physiology)
3. Spiritual (mental/emotional)

Your ultimate health is achieved by maintaining a harmonious balance of these three aspects. Accumulation of environmental toxins (such as those from heavy metals, pollution, drugs, and processed foods) and endotoxins (stress hormones, tissue acidity, and digestive imbalances) will lead to chronic biochemical dysfunction and ultimately accelerated aging. There are several theories of aging, including "Programmed Cell Death," which hypothesizes that cells have a finite life span for cell division leading to eventual cell death. Based upon this theory, the hypothetical upper limit for the human lifespan may be as high as one hundred and twenty years.

Then why don't we all live to be a hundred and twenty? Dr. Denham Harmon proposed the "free radical theory of aging" in 1954. He hypothesized that "free radicals," which are highly charged, unstable molecular fragments (from metabolism, toxins, radiation, etc.) naturally generated in our bodies, cause oxidation and cellular breakdown. Therefore, if a person's free radical load is too high, it causes accelerated destruction of cell membranes, disrupts key enzyme systems, and fractures DNA. This will ultimately compromise many body systems, including the immune system, cellular and organ repair, and energy production. This process may result in a myriad of degenerative conditions including fatigue, infections, allergies, and autoimmune diseases such as arthritis, multiple sclerosis, and cancer.

This "free radical overload" contributes to systemic disruption, and the resulting chronic diseases have a major impact on shortening our potential lifespan of a hundred and twenty years to an average expectation of seventy-five to eighty-five years in North America. A prime example is if you are a smoker with diabetes and high blood pressure and don't look after yourself, by the chronological age of fifty, you may have had enough accumulated damage to your organs and body functions that you are experiencing accelerated aging. Due to this damage, you may be "biologically aged" closer to seventy-five or eighty, and you could therefore die of old age at a chronological age of only fifty or fifty-five.

To slow or decelerate cellular aging, one must embrace the concept of "metabolic detoxification". This process assists in the elimination of toxins and metabolic by-products in your body and the reduction of free-radical oxidation. The goal is to reduce your toxic load through a healthy, balanced diet; regular, effective exercise; nutritional (antioxidant) support; and optimal hormone balancing in order to have optimal systemic and body functions leading to a long and healthy life full of vitality.

Another significant and effective "anti-aging" intervention is the use of "hormone optimization". From the time when we were children and through our teenage years, the sexual hormones in our bodies were primarily there for growth and development. Later, through our twenties, thirties, and forties, these same hormones were there with and added emphasis on human reproduction. Beyond the "fertile child bearing period," our bodies move naturally into menopause and andropause (male menopause). At this time, your physiology is saying, "OK, we're not reproducing anymore, we're not growing any more, so let's concentrate on using the hormones for body repair." In a global biological sense, if one is past the childrearing stage and is no longer reproducing, one is now considered biologically expendable, and the progress toward accelerated physiological aging and death is emphasized. This "degenerative aging process" is in large part due to a significantly lowered hormone baseline production in the "elderly" - as evidenced by baseline sexual hormone levels at only a fraction of "youthful baseline hormone levels."

When your hormones are reduced significantly, your body's natural regenerative mechanisms become less efficient, and your ability to repair damaged or diseased tissues is greatly diminished. A classic example of this is when a child falls and scrapes his/her knee, it may take three days to heal, but when you're fifty-five and suffer a similar trauma, it may take you two or more weeks to fully heal. That's an example of your body losing its ability to repair efficiently and hence the beginning of the degenerative process.

The hormone/endocrine system is therefore extremely important to the body's regeneration potential - it is in essence the heart of the "anti-aging" process within our bodies. Endo (internally generated) and exo (externally generated) toxins that generate an excess of cell-damaging free radicals are the primary obstacles to and disruptors of this regenerative system and therefore prevent it from doing its job.

The following is a very important question: What is your toxic load, and where are your toxins coming from? Removing toxins and reducing your total toxic burden is one of the most effective ways to restore your health and slow down aging. The first step is to assess and eliminate toxins in the body. What are these toxins, and how can we prevent having them accumulate in our bodies?

Here are some potential toxic sources:

- Indoor pollution: household cleaning products, mold, dust, and carpeting
- Environmental pollution: exhaust, smoke, and poor oxygen levels.
- Chemicals in food, water, personal care products, pesticides
- Radiation, noise pollution, heavy metals (mercury, lead, aluminum, cadmium)
- Pharmacological and non-pharmacological drugs such as caffeine and alcohol
- Diet: Trans fats, sugar, food coloring, additives, preservatives
- Allergies: Foods, dust, mold, airborne, seasonal, pollution, animal dander
- Chronic infections: Yeasts, bacteria, viruses, and parasites
- Nutritional deficiencies: Nutrient-poor foods, processed foods, and foods low in essential fatty acids, vitamins and minerals, or digestive enzymes
- Metabolic imbalances: Gut flora, chronic inflammation, dysfunctional organ systems (poor elimination), and hormonal imbalance/dysfunction
- Psycho-emotional: Lack of joy or purpose, isolation, fear, overwork

and exhaustion, poor sleep, loneliness, poor self-esteem, pessimism, feelings of powerlessness
- Lack of adequate and proper exercise
- Spiritual: Lack of trust in self and others, feeling separated from nature, and little sense of connection to the universe or a higher meaning in life

Our bodies have an amazing capacity to adapt and function under emotional and environmental stress for long periods of time. But chronic stress both internal and external may result in an excessive accumulation of toxic elements, and it is this total toxic burden that ultimately leads to cellular/organ degeneration and failure. An example of this is that at age twenty, you may have a relatively low level of toxicity, but by the time you hit age forty or fifty, the total toxic burden has increased while your hormones have already started their natural decline. This confluence of factors exert tremendous pressure on one's physiology, resulting in the start of accelerated aging and chronic poor health.

Endotoxins are naturally occurring toxic chemicals that occur inside our bodies as a result of normal metabolic processes. For example, metabolic waste by-products are produced when we eat and digest food. If the system is healthy, the body will extract the nutrients from your food and eliminate the metabolic toxins. But if your elimination system (such as the digestive tract) is disrupted, toxins accumulate, and your overall toxic burden rises and can disrupt the healthy function of other bodily systems.

In North America, our dietary habits and food choices are usually nutrient poor and overly processed. This coupled with compromised healthy elimination results in an increasing toxic burden. This is a vicious cycle with increasing toxic load negatively impacting successful elimination and neutralization of toxins. The perfect storm of impaired body repair and toxic accumulation is a disastrous combination.

It is, therefore, crucial that before any hormone therapies have a chance to be successful, you must adequately eliminate body toxins. The majority of therapies targeting cognitive and systemic enhancement are all predicated on how efficient your body physiology is in terms of being able to cleanse and to renew itself. You want your body to be an empty canvas. You want to start fresh and stay fresh. Simplicity is very important.

Our ancestors had a lifestyle that consisted of eating simple home-cooked meals during the week punctuated with a communal feast on the weekends. In modern society, however, our diet has become more complex, and we eat out more often and have daily feasts punctuated by weekend super-feasts.

Our bodies cannot sustain this overindulgence. Over time, this over-consumption and food complexity elevates metabolic toxins in the body. Weight gain and obesity are significant health problems in Western. Those afflicted feel fatigued and experience sore joints and muscles as inflammation rises. For the average overweight sedentary North American, by the time you're forty years old, your blood sugar is too high, and you are overweight (high BMI) and gaining additional weight every year. Your sleep is compromised, and your hair is prematurely graying and falling out. All of this may occur due to the heavy accumulation of metabolic toxins that accelerate aging and promote chronic degenerative diseases.

Signs and symptoms of toxicity:
- Sensitivity to chemicals, car fumes, odors, perfumes
- Increasingly affected by caffeine, alcohol, or medications
- Sensitivity to foods with sulfites, such as wine, dried fruits or soda
- Fibromyalgia, chronic fatigue syndrome, cancer, or autoimmune disease
- Skin prone to eczema, hives, or acne

- Sore joints, muscle aches, fatigue, or weakness
- Mood swings, irritability, or anxiety
- A lack of concentration, focus, or motivation
- Loss of libido and sexual function
- Frequent colds and infections with slow recovery time
- Bad breath or foul-smelling bowel movements
- Chronically bloated and gaseous
- Frequent headaches, sinus congestion, allergies, or infections
- Lackluster, dry, and prematurely wrinkled skin
- Early head hair loss

These can all be indicators of toxins in your body. Some of them are part of aging, but we always want to have a lower biological age versus chronological age – to be chronological age fifty but to look and feel a younger thirty. Most people are unfortunately the other way around, but you can look and feel younger by taking care of yourself by identifying and reducing your toxic burden.

The first step towards optimizing your health is to assess what toxins you are exposed to and your current toxic burden. This inventory will allow you to become more aware and educated as to what is needed to reduce your toxic burden.

Make a checklist of how you feel. Are my joints sore? Am I tired in the mornings? Is my diet healthy? Am I eating too much junk food? Am I eating on time? Am I drinking enough water? Am I taking too many medicines or drugs? Is there too much stress in my life? Is my household too dusty, moldy, or toxic? Am I happy? Do I have love in my life? Start by looking at the list and working backward. You need to go through your house and eliminate toxic items.

Use less-toxic elements in your skin creams, cosmetics, soaps, and shampoos. You will want to implement the use of water filters. Drinking pure water is critical. Make sure chlorine, environmental chemicals, and heavy metals are cleared from your drinking water. Also, consider showerhead filters that are effective in eliminating vaporized chlorine. Assessing your body's heavy metal burden for mercury, lead, cadmium, and aluminum can be a very important step towards optimal health. The toxic heavy metals can have a devastating effect on many of the body systems. They can harm your neurological, digestive, cardiovascular, immune, and reproductive systems, including the hormones that help repair cells and organs. These heavy metals can be accumulated through exposure from dental amalgam fillings, paints, glazing, vinyl products, pollution, food (especially seafood), and medicine. To determine your heavy metal levels, you may need to do specialized lab testing. It is essential to reduce these levels if the burden is significant in order to decrease cellular aging and optimize health and vitality.

What to Eat and Why

Eating simply and without excess is the key. Eat a diet that favors natural, unprocessed, organic foods that don't have a lot of pesticides or additives. You want to eat as many things as you can that have good, healthy antioxidants. Eat food that's fresh and in season as much as possible.

Fewer animal proteins are better. Our bodies are omnivorous, so I don't believe you need to be totally vegetarian. I think that the majority of people do better with a small quantity of animal protein while consuming more fruits and vegetables. Eat a "rainbow diet" comprised of carotene-rich foods with color such as peppers, carrots, radishes, and leafy green vegetables. These foods also have higher amounts of lycopene, are nutrient rich, and have high levels of antioxidants.

You can also eat healthy fats found in nuts like almonds, pecans, walnuts, and cashews. They provide desirable fats, nutrients, and cell protection. Wild salmon is also high in Omega 3 oil, which is another healthy fat.

Berries are antioxidant and nutrient rich. Acai berries are considered to be a "super food," and research shows that they have a high oxygen radical absorption capacity (ORAC value). The antioxidant properties of the berries effectively neutralize harmful free radicals in your body. Other good antioxidant sources are berries such as strawberries, blueberries, bilberries, and pomegranate – eat them organic.

Juicing organic fruits and vegetables is another excellent way to introduce these "super-foods" into your daily diet. Green tea is another great beverage choice. It can assist in weight control and protects against oxidation and inflammation. If you are tolerant to dairy, kefir (a fermented milk drink) and yogurt can also provide excellent sources of nutrition and probiotics for healthy gastrointestinal function.

Also in the "should-eat" category are foods high in chlorophyll, which is found in leafy green plants. Vegetables such as broccoli, spinach, kale, spirulina, onions, peppers, sprouts, avocados, and tomatoes contain abundant phytochemicals that are loaded with fiber and chlorophyll, which are nutrients that protect the cells of your body. Chlorophyll helps keep the intestinal tract healthy. When your intestinal tract is healthy, it will help your body reduce its toxic burden, eliminate properly, and keep your cells revitalized. Your body is then able to effectively absorb additional nutrients.

As far as taking vitamin supplements, it's the usual suspects: the B vitamins and Vitamin E (take a complex E). I also like to use glutathione. It's an amino acid that is a super antioxidant produced in your liver. It grabs free radicals and neutralizes them and also helps the body build up a better oxygen capacity and improves immune system function. One of the best new supplements is a super antioxidant called resveratrol, which is made from the skin of red grapes and has been clinically shown to protect against cardiovascular disease and degenerative diseases such as cancer.

Get Rid of Toxins

If you need more guidance on your diet, you should contact a health professional that is well educated in practical clinical nutrition such as a naturopathic physician. The key underlying principle is to restore the vital organ systems to optimal functional capacity, thereby favoring body system repair and decelerated cellular aging.

These four organ systems are of primary importance in the elimination of metabolic toxicity.

The Liver

The liver is key in digestion and elimination of nutrients and waste products. Your liver is critical for helping your body process hormones. Alcohol, processed foods, and drugs can burden it. If you take too many drugs like Tylenol, painkillers, and anti-inflammatories, your liver gets plugged up. The things you can take to help your liver are glutathione, Vitamin C, milk thistle, senna leaves, and cascara. These all help dump toxins and get your liver moving.

Kidneys

The kidneys filter and eliminate waste products through the urine while maintaining healthy acid/base balance in our connective tissue and blood. When your body's acidity goes up in the connective tissues, your body is burdened and has to dump the acid. Organic acids create joint problems and inflammation, producing many kinds of degenerative conditions such as cancer, arthritis, and eczema. Make sure that your kidneys are filtering efficiently, and assist them by drinking an adequate amount of water and taking cleansing herbs like goldenrod and bilberry.

Gastro-intestinal Tract

A healthy small and large bowel is essential for digestion, nutrient extraction, and elimination of waste products. Poor bowel function results in autointoxication and chronic health issues. If your digestive tract is not moving, it may have impacted fecal matter. If you're not eliminating properly, you are going to be reabsorbing toxins you should be eliminating. To assist, you should drink enough water (a minimum of 1 to 1.5 liters of filtered and alkalized water per day) and eat enough fiber. Fiber is in brown flax seeds and psyllium. Chlorophyll – which is be found in spirulina, seaweed, and the green foods mentioned before – is also important for the digestive tract. Probiotics – bacteria like acidophilus – can be helpful as well.

Respiratory System/Lungs

Another way to effectively eliminate body toxins is through the lungs. We breathe in fresh air and breathe out stale air, including carbonic acid. This system also helps reduce stress and keeps our body from building up excess acidity. Exercises like Yoga and Tai Chi focus our breath work on deep breathing. Deep breathing allows your body to regenerate by adding fresh air and has the added bonus of relieving stress.

Another simple way to detox the body is through a fasting diet to eliminate any foods to which you might be sensitive or allergic. Classic detoxification diets specifically used to reduce toxic load and promote gastrointestinal health include alkaline-favored diets, non-wheat/gluten diets, elimination diets, candida or parasitic-elimination diets, and lower glycemic-index diets, to name a few.

In Summary

"Genes load the gun, the environment pulls the trigger." It is the removal of these environmental toxins that prevents the genes from having to act and cause disease. The longer we live, the more toxins and heavy metals we have in our tissue, and the more they affect our health; therefore, before we can successfully implement anti-aging medicine, we need to assess and reduce our metabolic toxic burden that disrupts our physiology.

Body system dysfunction will result in poor health and disease. Stress also contributes significantly to our toxic load. Reducing these poisons allows our natural repair systems to minimize premature cellular aging.

FELICIA PIZZONIA, R.H.N

There is a need for an integrative approach to age management, which includes the identification and elimination of metabolic toxic burden through lifestyle, diet, exercise, hormone optimization, and structural and psycho-emotional balancing. This is a critical component of any effective anti-aging strategy that is directed towards the goal of attaining optimal health, vitality, and longevity.

Dr. Lawrence Chan

Dr. Chan has a strong personal interest in preventative, functional, and anti-aging medicine in the fullest sense: the health of mind, body, and spirit.

Dr. Chan grew up watching his father, uncle, and their colleagues practice Tai Chi and traditional Chinese medicine. His ambition was to follow in his father's footsteps. He studied martial arts from a young age, and in addition to learning lessons of perseverance and patience, he learned how the flow of energy in our body universally affects health and vitality.

Dr. Chan earned his bachelor's degree from Simon Fraser University in Canada and his doctorate at the Canadian Memorial Chiropractic College. He also has doctorates in naturopathic medicine and traditional Chinese acupuncture.

Dr. Chan has successfully created, with his business partners, one of the largest integrated health facilities in Canada – the Integrative Healing Arts Centre in Vancouver, British Columbia. This multi-disciplinary center was established in 1985 and includes an integrative naturopathic spa for aesthetic and restorative age management.

Dr. Lawrence Chan
Integrative Healing Arts
Suite 730, 1285 W. Broadway
Vancouver, British Columbia, Canada
V6H 3X8

Phone: 604-738-1012
E-mail: info@integrative.ca
www.integrative.ca

CHAPTER THREE

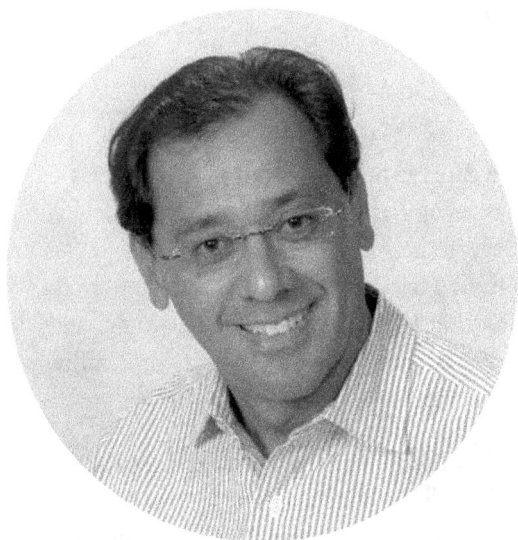

Dr. David Garcia:

Inflammation

CHAPTER THREE

Dr. David Garcia: Inflammation

Before I explain how inflammation can lead to problems that can hasten aging, let me tell you what I feel you should know. I believe that if an idea, situation, or goal is created in our minds, the simple fact that it was planted there makes it possible to achieve. I think that God places noble ideas there and He wants us to proceed with confidence, knowing that there is a divine purpose and direction behind these ideas.

The writer and philosopher Henry David Thoreau said it best: "If one advances confidently in the direction of his dreams, and endeavors to live the life which he has imagined, he will meet with a success unexpected in common hours." As long as you can dream it, you can do it. I also believe that we are superior to any circumstance in which we find ourselves – even when the situation is the natural process of aging.

My life's path has proven these statements to be true. I am a first-generation American and the youngest of four children born to a Presbyterian minister. I was influenced to become a doctor by an uncle who was the first physician in my extended family. I remember, as a young child, being mesmerized by his stories of the hospital, his radiology practice, and its challenges. I was influenced as well by my older brother and sister, who also became physicians (before me) after hearing our uncle's tales.

I graduated medical school in 1989 and went into a primary care residency. For more than twenty years, I've worked in emergency rooms, urgent care, and primary care as well as performed aesthetic services and anti-aging services.

Over time and as I gained experience, I began to re-evaluate how traditional medicine is practiced. I noticed that ER and urgent care treatment was episodic, that is, a person was treated for a particular illness only to return later and have to be treated again for that exact same illness. I wondered if there was another way to produce long-lasting and profound changes. I began to attend anti-aging conferences sponsored by the American Academy of Anti-aging Medicine. I took a fellowship to train in functional and regenerative medicine.

After reviewing many theories of aging, what became of particular interest to me were the changes produced by hormone optimization along with pharmaceutical nutrients and exercise. I felt that I'd stumbled onto some profound knowledge and was determined to practice this type of medicine.

It's been postulated by medical experts that chronic inflammation is the cause and effect of illness and the diseases of aging. The downtick of human vitality generally begins in our forties. With the average lifespan in the United States reaching more than seventy-eight years in 2010, far outpacing the world average of sixty-six years (according to the CIA), that's a lot of years in which you need to keep yourself healthy and active!

What is inflammation? There are two main types. The first type, acute inflammation, is the body's response to injury, infection, or stress. Inflammatory mediators called cytokines are released and show the classical signs of inflammation: swelling, redness, heat, pain, and loss of function. This type of inflammation will subside once the injury, illness, or stress is removed and the body has healed itself.

The second, silent inflammation, occurs when one or more of the triggers do not go away. This causes the excessive production of cytokines, which are protein molecules secreted by cells of the immune system that regulate it. It's called silent because it cannot be felt.

It's this second type that is associated with many of the degenerative diseases of aging. Silent inflammation is caused by the production of a type of hormone called eicosanoids. They are signal molecules that are made by the oxidation of twenty carbon essential fatty acids. They exert control over many bodily systems, mainly in inflammation or immunity, and act as messengers for the central nervous system.

There are pro-inflammatory eicosanoids that can cause tissue destruction over time. Eicosanoids are increased by the type of diet a person eats but mainly by ingestion of omega-6 fatty acids. Also associated with silent inflammation are high levels of insulin, cortisol, abdominal fat, and normal aging.

I understand that the true cause of many aging syndromes come from silent inflammation. If left unchecked, this silent inflammation can cause debilitating disease. Low-level chronic inflammation is associated with all the classic diseases of old age in addition to loss of muscle mass and strength. These diseases and conditions include heart disease, type 2 diabetes, decreased cognitive function, Alzheimer's, rheumatoid arthritis, lupus, autoimmune disease, cancer, osteoporosis, metabolic syndrome, stress, obesity, and declining hormone levels.

Silent inflammation can be detected and measured easily with the analysis of blood work. By using very easy methods of cytokine-lowering treatment, many degenerative diseases of aging can be suppressed. The trick is to treat all these diverse conditions "upstream" before they even start (though they can certainly be treated well even after they start) for a long, healthy, vibrant life with full cognitive control.

This treatment "for life" includes finding the best diet and herbal and vitamin supplements for each person along with hormone optimization.

How can you combat inflammation? There are several supplements that can be used. They include high-grade fish oil; curcumin; olive oil; the vitamins B, C, D, E, and K; Coenzyme Q10; beta-carotene (a precursor to vitamin A); alpha lipoic acid; n-acetyl cysteine; green tea extract; grape seed extract; resveratrol; and carnosine. There are also hormone supplements that decrease inflammation, and they include DHEA, testosterone, estrogen, thyroid, and growth hormone.

In addition to supplements and hormone therapy, there are foods that prevent silent inflammation by reducing high levels of insulin. Insulin increases arachidonic acid, which is the precursor to pro-inflammatory eicosanoids. These whole foods have a low value on the glycemic index. They include fruits and vegetables, egg whites, canned tuna, lean meats in portions approximately the size of the palm of your hand, and low-fat cottage cheese. All processed carbohydrates and anything high in sugar should be removed from your diet to reduce the glycemic load on your body.

After my training and study, I co-founded BodyLogicMD of Columbus, Ohio, an anti-aging firm with an emphasis on bioidentical hormones, nutrition, and fitness. Bioidentical hormones are molecular messengers in the body that regulate many processes in the body. When we are in our twenties, these hormones are most optimized. With time and age, they do steadily go down, and we have less energy, less sleep, less reserves, less focus, less libido, more aches and pains, more irritability, and more couch-potato mentality. Optimizing these bioidentical hormones to youthful levels can reverse these symptoms. The results I've seen so far have just been amazing! I think we are on the cusp of a revolution regarding how medicine is practiced. I believe that there will be an even greater number of new life extension therapies in the near future.

I have seen great turnarounds in health and vitality with my patients, my family, and even myself using these techniques. My 89-year-old father is vibrant, cognizant, funny, and insightful. He was definitely less active and less physically powerful before treatment to reduce his inflammation and increase his bioidentical hormones. He had been feeling weaker and weaker especially since he walked with a walker due to a stroke more than twenty years ago. He walks well, he travels a lot, he's currently writing his memoirs, and he has a forceful opinion, especially when it comes to politics. He states he will never stop the therapy because he wants to continue to feel good and be active and not go under the "decline."

There is a quantum level of difference in patient outcomes when my techniques are used early for prevention and optimization rather than treating the vast array of different diseases "downstream." Traditional medicine is focused on the downstream (after it happens), whereas my colleagues and I are focused upstream (in prevention). My hope and dream is that the rest of the medical field will cease to be reactionary and will soon follow our path to good health and a longer, more active life.

Dr. David Garcia

Dr. David Garcia is a leading osteopathic doctor with more than twenty years of experience. His expertise is also in demand in the fields of anti-aging, family, occupational, addiction, and emergency medicine.

Dr. Garcia is a first-generation American and the youngest of four born in Corsicana, Texas, after his parents moved there in the early 1950s to seek a better life. After graduating high school, Dr. Garcia attended Ohio State University and the Ohio University College of Osteopathic Medicine. He did his primary care residency at Richmond Heights General Hospital in Cleveland. Dr. Garcia has treated addicted patients at the Suboxone Clinic of Columbus and is also an independent medical examiner.

With his brother (also a physician), Dr. Garcia co-founded an urgent care center. In addition, he opened an aesthetics and an anti-aging company to accommodate patients and their ongoing needs. BodyLogicMD, the anti-aging firm, is based in Columbus, Ohio, and emphasizes the use of hormones, nutrition, and fitness for health. He's also a consultant for NHT Global, where he helps develop ideas for new anti-aging products.

When not practicing medicine, Dr. Garcia loves spending time with his wife, Dru, and sons Roman, six, and Preston, three. Before the birth of his sons, Dr. Garcia went scuba diving with sharks, ran with bulls in Pamplona, and traveled extensively. He can't wait until they get a little older and will be able to go on these adventures together. Mt. Kilimanjaro awaits!

Dr. David Garcia
BodyLogicMD of Columbus
Suite 100, 1120 Polaris Parkway
Columbus, Ohio, United States
43240

Phone: 888-657-4562
E-mail: drdavidgarcia@yahoo.com

CHAPTER FOUR

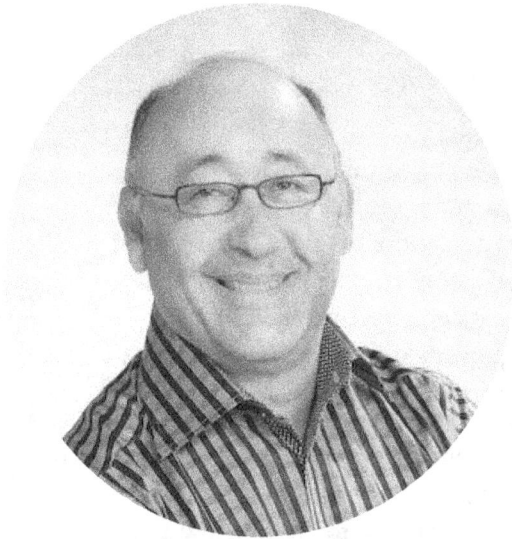

Dr. Roger Garcia:

Adrenal Fatigue

CHAPTER FOUR

Dr. Roger Garcia: Adrenal Fatigue

I
t's my belief that inferior doctors treat disease, and superior physicians prevent it. I see patients come to the hospital who are dying from conditions that could have been prevented, from things that could have been treated early and never were. As an emergency room doctor, I developed an interest in anti-aging therapies from seeing these patients who were getting sicker and sicker and dying in their early forties.

Part of the problem is with modern medicine's focus on seeing patients in a very short period of time in the ER – about 15 minutes each – which is not enough time to get to know a person before prescribing them medicine. It's about turning out patients as quickly as possible to make money.

And that's not the kind of doctor I wanted to be. I always knew I wanted to be a doctor, but in the real world, the romance and ideal of spending time and caring for patients individually got lost as I found myself becoming caught up in the stress of running a practice and the business side of medicine. It gets to you after a while, and I developed hypocortisolism, otherwise known as adrenal dysfunction or more commonly known as adrenal fatigue.

The adrenal glands are small endocrine organs located on the top of each kidney. They are probably the most important endocrine glands in the body. Their purpose is to respond to every stress in your life: mental, emotional, environmental, and physical. These adrenal glands shoot out various hormones—cortisol, aldosterone, pregnenolone, progesterone, and DHEA from the cortex and epinephrine and norepinephrine from the medulla—all designed to help you deal with the stresses of everyday life. Without these hormones, you wouldn't be able to function.

The main player in this adrenal milieu is cortisol, as it is used to optimize human performance. It allows us to function optimally at work, at play, and during athletic contests, and it also alerts us to danger. It gets us prepared for the "fight or flight" response by making the heart beat faster and contract more strongly, increasing blood pressure, and increasing blood sugar levels to provide strength and energy. This has the effect of providing an increased amount of oxygen and nutrients to specific areas of the body needed in such an emergency. It also is involved in many other things. It stimulates appetite; regulates the metabolism of proteins, carbohydrates, and fats; slows the immune system's inflammatory response that helps with pain; improves digestion; eases movement in the joints; soothes allergies, fever, and reactions to toxins; and enhances the immune system.

Whether our stress comes from athletic performance or from deadlines at work, our body sends out cortisol to help us deal with it.

But our world and its toxins are affecting everything about us. The toxins are everywhere: from the air we breathe to the water we drink and the food we eat, which is processed, genetically modified, and filled with chemical and artificial ingredients like Sucralose.

The problem is that we're so inundated with stresses and toxins in our lives today that our adrenal glands are under constant demand and never get a chance to slow down and recover. In a normal stress reaction, the sympathetic nervous system activates the hypothalamic-pituitary-adrenal (HPA) axis. Corticotropin-releasing hormone (CRH) from the hypothalamus induces adrenocorticotropin (ACTH) release from the pituitary that signals the adrenal cortex to release the glucocorticoid, cortisol, and the androgen, dihydroepiandosterone (DHEA). These stress hormones are two sides of the same coin in a normal stress reaction. That is, the increase of cortisol is catabolic ("eating away"), causing the breakdown of stored glycogen, protein, and fats to produce glucose for the "fight or flight" response. This increase in cortisol will inhibit further release of ACTH by a negative feedback loop, thereby moderating the stress response when it is short-lived. DHEA is the anabolic side ("rebuilding side") of the stress reaction further moderating the stress response by rebuilding tissue when the stress response is short-lived. However, it is the unrelenting demand upon the adrenal gland through physical, environmental, physiological, and mental stressors over time in twenty-first century man that eventually leads to a reduction in the output of cortisol and DHEA that is the hallmark of adrenal fatigue. The allostatic load ("wear and tear") of these various stressors will impact the degree of adrenal dysfunction we live with. When you add to this prolonged stress reaction the natural reduction of our DHEA levels of 2 percent per year as a result of aging, catabolic activity will increase over anabolic activity, leading to the development of a host of chronic disease states by different mechanisms, including the reduction of all of our hormones.

The loss of DHEA means that catabolism reigns, thereby leading to decreased glucose utilization, elevated blood glucose levels, and eventually insulin resistance. This has the effect of adding pounds, particularly around the belly. Eventually, metabolic syndrome will arise from this central obesity, leading to diabetes and hypertension with damage to blood vessels and the development of arthrosclerosis. Without intervention, the risk of cardiovascular disease (heart attack) and cerebral vascular disease (stroke) rises.

In addition, the mineralcorticoid, aldosterone, found in the adrenal cortex is also affected by adrenal fatigue. It is a hormone that regulates minerals and salts in the body and thereby stabilizes blood pressure. Adrenal fatigue will result in low blood pressure with dizzy spells or feelings of wooziness when standing.

As doctors, we like to evaluate individual hormones as a way to quantify them and get a handle on disease states. The truth is they are all interdependent on each other so that when one is out of whack, it produces profound effects on the other hormones. This also is true among body systems. That is, the adrenal does not function in isolation when it comes to the response to prolonged stress. There is continuous cross-talk and stress-induced imbalances among the central nervous system (imbalances of neurotransmitters), the immune system (imbalances of cytokines), the digestive system (leaky gut), and the endocrine system (hormone imbalance), with each system's response to stress having an impact on the others.

For example, repeated stress leads to hypercortisolism and brain function degeneration, particularly the hippocampus losing the ability to repair itself (the hypothalamus, pre-frontal cortex, and amygdala can also be involved). Because the hippocampus has a large concentration of cortisol receptors, it serves to regulate the response of the HPA axis to stress by regulating the hypothalamus (it's the on-and-off switch for the hypothalamus). With progressive degeneration of the hippocampus to prolonged stress, it can no longer inhibit the hypothalamus, leading to an increased cortisol response and more oxidative stress that further accelerates hippocampus degeneration. Because the hippocampus is the memory center of the brain, its degeneration will lead to impaired memory, dementia, and depression. Eventually, with continued prolonged stress, cortisol levels will flatten with resulting immune system microglia activation leading to an increase in the pro-inflammatory cytokine molecules (tumor necrosis factor alpha and interleukin 6) with subsequent immune inflammation. This will lead to serotonin degradation and eventually to stage III adrenal exhaustion with a flattened cortisol response to further stressors. The immune system dysfunction causes elevations of immune mediators, causing body-wide inflammation that is the source of such disparate disease states ranging from cardiovascular disease, dysbiosis, autoimmune states, chronic fatigue, and fibromyalgia to such mood disorders as bipolar disorder, schizophrenia, and depression.

The first step in reversing this deteriorating cascade of events is to ensure the ability to reach phase three and four slow wave sleep that allows for neurogenesis (growth of new brain cells) through release of growth hormone and melatonin and reversal of inflammation mediated by the immune system.

The endocrine system will also have many imbalances in various hormones stemming from the prolonged stress reaction. The steroidogenic pathway that produces much of our sex and adrenal hormones begins with cholesterol. This pathway will predominately be shifted toward the production of cortisol with chronic stress, resulting in a reduction of all of our hormones. This is in addition to the increase of cortisol that occurs with the aging process itself even in a non stressed person. It's a circular downward pattern.

The production of testosterone for men and women begins to diminish; women also begin to lose progesterone and estrogen. With the loss of progesterone and estrogen in women, good quality sleep becomes a by-gone memory. The inability to sleep leads again to more weight gains and stress. Sleep disturbance leads to inconsistent melatonin production, with resulting further loss of sleep. The reduction of this most powerful anti-oxidant and the pro-oxidant effect of sleeplessness predispose women to a higher risk of breast cancer and men to a higher risk of prostate cancer. Women who can't sleep often gain eight to ten pounds because of the amount of insulin resistance they develop with pro-inflammatory molecules made within the increased fat cells crossing the blood-brain barrier, leading to depression and igniting further stress and inflammation within the immune system. The hypocortisolism that results is postulated to be one mechanism that results in high mortality and increased metastasis in women diagnosed with breast cancer.

In addition, this inflammatory state interferes with the function of leptin. Leptin is a hormone made within fat cells that signals the brain there are adequate energy stores (fat), suppresses our appetite, and speeds up our metabolism. The leptin resistance that ensues further stresses us by leading to more weight gain and therefore more inflammation and the negative downward cycle grows.

Increased cortisol disrupts the metabolism of estrogen. The insulin resistance with increased cortisol that ensues leads to more androgen production and subsequent conversion of these androgens to estrogen within the ever-growing fat cells. Estrogen elimination through the gut and phase II detoxification in the liver is disrupted by this elevated cortisol.

In men, as a result of the decreased production of testosterone, insulin resistance increases, as testosterone's natural antagonistic properties to the stress hormones have also decreased in tandem with the loss of testosterone. Weight gain around the belly becomes commonplace, and a cycle of decreasing testosterone begins by the conversion of testosterone to estrogen by the enzyme aromatase found within the fat cells. The inflammatory cascade that develops along with the rising proportion of estrogen increases clotting factors and narrowing of the coronary arteries, leading to an escalating risk of heart attacks and strokes.

Stress also suppresses growth hormone. And as growth hormone diminishes, you have aches and pains, an increase in body fat, and a loss of concentration.

The metabolic hormones in the thyroid also diminish; the activation of CRH and glucocorticoids from stress will lead to hypothyroidism by two mechanisms. First, they will inhibit TSH (thyroid-stimulating hormone) directly, causing a drop off in thyroid hormone and resulting slowdown in metabolism. They will also inhibit the conversion of T4 to T3. This conversion is critical, as it is T3 that is the active metabolite responsible for a robust metabolism. Instead of T3, the inactive reverse T3 is made from T4 as a compensatory mechanism to stress caused by the mistaken perception by the body that it is functioning in a famine state. As a result, metabolism slows to preserve calories, but the net effect is a functional hypothyroid state. Here again we see the development of increased weight gain with all of its inflammation, in addition to the hallmarks of hypothyroidism including concentration and focus issues, hair loss, and elevated cholesterol values. This hypothyroid condition will be missed by those following just the TSH, as it will be normal or low due to this inhibition (free T4, free T3, and reverse T3 must also be checked to ensure this does not happen). Supplementing with zinc and selenium will help correct this reverse T3 condition and should be the first course of action prior to supplementing with thyroid medications.

Giving thyroid supplementation in the face of this functional hypothyroid condition caused by prolonged stress will cause one to feel much worse. The adrenals must be supported first for two or three months in an effort to get them back on track prior to thyroid medication. Failure to do so will increase metabolism without the adrenal reserve to keep up, and the resulting stress will exponentially compound their fatigued condition.

The slow loss of cortisol reduces the amount of cortisol receptors in the body, lessens the sensitivity of the receptors, and decreases the amount of tryptophan available to make serotonin. Serotonin is a neurotransmitter that helps with your feelings of well-being. It regulates mood, appetite, sleep, memory, and learning. Without serotonin, you end up feeling chronically fatigued. This down-regulation leads to a decrease in our ability to mount a stress response and is speculated to be a protective mechanism by our bodies against the ravages of stress.

As you can imagine, a person who has adrenal dysfunction feels like a shell of his or her former self. He or she has mental problems; sleep difficulties leading to mood, memory, focus, and concentration difficulties in addition to weight gain; aches and pains; anxiousness; fatigue; blood-pressure problems; and a greater risk of infections and allergies.

It's a devastating condition that will ultimately lay the groundwork for developing more troublesome problems like cancer. But before then, you'll be hitting all the other degenerative diseases related to insulin resistance and obesity.

All of us have some measure of adrenal dysfunction because of our time-limited, stressful lifestyles that over time leave no time for play, recuperation, exercise, or preparation of good, nutritious, organic meals. We eventually get trapped in a downward spiral, as this adrenal dysfunction will lead to such fatigue that even participation in these activities is impossible without some intervention to improve adrenal functioning.

This adrenal dysfunction can be found in the gray area between conventional medicine's high cortisol condition, Cushing's syndrome, and the extremely low cortisol condition known as Addison's disease. But in the middle, there's a tremendous amount of adrenal dysfunction that is unrecognized but can be found if you know where to look. Research has established that measuring cortisol levels through a four-point saliva test is the gold standard. It can help us distinguish dysfunction of the diurnal pattern of cortisol that is not found using conventional medicine's all-or-nothing approach (high or low) when measuring cortisol. In fact, it has been demonstrated that plasma cortisol immunoassays are significantly inaccurate, overestimating serum cortisol levels by an average of 70 percent and resulting in the misclassification of 44-56 percent of patients. As well, urinary cortisol assays lack sensitivity due to the wide individual variations in cortisol excretion over twenty-four hours and do not tell us cortisol fluctuations throughout the day.

How do we address this "unseen" adrenal dysfunction to improve one's quality of life? First, one must engage in practices that will help reduce or manage the sympathetic trigger that brings on the stress response. Lifestyle modification is the buzzword. You should regularly participate in physical activity that you love because exercise lowers cortisol levels by increasing the "feel good hormones" dopamine and serotonin, in addition to the "runner's high," created by increased endorphin levels. You will gain muscle, strength, and bone density. It will protect against heart disease, colds, dementia, hot flashes, gum disease, diabetes, excess body fat, and depression. It supports your immune system; improves sleep; protects your bones, joints, and vision; and improves wound healing, sex, job performance, and the prospects of career advancement. What this all adds up to is less overall stress to the body and healthier recovery from the stress we all encounter on a daily basis.

The mind-body connection also can't be discounted. We have to surround ourselves with an epigenetic, self-nurturing environment where we can better deal with our stress, create inner peace, and release the difficult memories trapped within our bodies. Practice using techniques such as meditation, prayer, optimism, a positive attitude, energy medicine (reiki, quantum touch, and therapeutic touch), energy psychology (emotional freedom technique), visualizations that are positive, acts of kindness and love, and spirituality. Other techniques include using music, dancing, laughter, bubble baths, massage, yoga, or saunas. Try the technique that works for you, as by doing so, you are activating the parasympathetic relaxation response over the sympathetic stress response. By activating this response, the vagus nerve is stimulated, which releases the feel-good neurotransmitter acetylcholine. It is this chemical that balances the stressful effects of adrenalin and cortisol from the sympathetic nervous system. It douses the molecular inflammatory wildfire brought about by adrenalin and cortisol through the calming, anti-inflammatory effect whenever the vagus nerve is stimulated. And the beauty is you are in control in activating this relaxation response with the ability to overtake the stressful events of your day that you cannot control. This control issue in of itself is very empowering and therefore very anti-inflammatory.

There are other strategies that are designed to support the adrenals in order to reduce its catabolic effect. They include the plant "adaptogens," so called because they balance the negative effects of cortisol. If cortisol is too high, they will help it go down, and if it's too low, they will help it rise. Used for thousands of years in ancient Chinese and Indian medicine, these adaptogens promote physiological resistance to stress, fatigue, trauma, and anxiety by reducing the sympathetic responses to stress via various mechanisms. They are segregated into adaptogen subclasses that include the triterpenes, the phenylpropanes, and the oxylipins. These include ashwaganda, holy basil, siberian ginseng, relora, rhodiola rosea, schisandra maca, licorice root, and Rg3, which supports healthy neurotransmitter function.

Herbal supplements are another strategy to support the adrenals. The amino acid L-theanine from green tea (contains 1-3 percent of theanine) has historically been used for its relaxing and anti-anxiety effects. It increases GABA (gamma-amino-butyric acid), reduces restlessness and insomnia, and increases alpha waves (meditative state). Phosphatidyl serine also helps blunt the chronic stress-induced HPA axis activation by dampening stress-induced ACTH and cortisol release.

There are adrenal glandular extracts without hormones that assist in adrenal gland self-repair by providing the raw material it needs to function. Originally researched in the 1940s, as potentially effective for altitude-induced adrenal stress in military pilots, they have been found to promote endogenous adrenal hormone production. They should, however, not be used as monotherapy for adrenal dysfunction but in combination with other nutritional strategies.

Additionally, certain vitamins and mineral nutrients are specifically used by the adrenals and therefore should be used to treat adrenal dysfunction. They include the use of magnesium (glycinate or citrate form), Vitamin C (2 to 5 grams daily), B vitamins (especially B5 up to 1.5 grams daily), selenium, zinc, calcium, copper, sodium, manganese, and Vitamin E with mixed tocopherols. Of note is that the adrenal glands are the organs in the body with the highest concentration of Vitamin C which is required for norepinephrine production. During periods of stress, the adrenal glands release Vitamin C within the gland locally, rather than systemically, to increase adrenal nitric oxide production, modify ACTH receptor sensitivity, and result in adrenal vascular vasodilatation. The net effect of these actions is to increase cortisol delivery while at the same time normalizing cortisol and ACTH levels.

The same dietary modifications you make to support your hormones also apply to the adrenals. We have the ability to modulate the inflammation within our bodies by changing the foods we eat. Whole foods, plant-based foods, seeds, fruits, vegetables, legumes, whole grains, and omega-3 fatty acids like fish oil are important. You should combine unrefined carbohydrates (whole grains) with good quality protein and oils (nuts and seeds) at most meals with small frequent meals throughout the day (using unrefined salt when needed). Use cold-pressed oils such as olive, walnut, filbert, and flax. In other words, ingestion of foods with anti-oxidant properties will help to reverse the free-radical damage caused by an inflammatory body. Foods that contain omega-6 fatty acids—such as trans fats and hydrogenated vegetable oils, refined carbohydrates, and junk foods—should be avoided along with caffeine, chocolate, and allergenic or sensitive foods.

Finally, in cases with severe adrenal dysfunction, pharmacologic agents can be used. Physiologic doses (15 mg) of hydrocortisone may be used while the adrenal is being supplemented but only for the shortest time possible. Unlike prednisone, these physiologic doses do not cause bone loss, adrenal suppression, or immune suppression. Hydrocortisone has been found to improve cellular and hormonal immunity and has been shown to be effective treatment in patients with chronic fatigue syndrome and fibromyalgia. In patients with orthostatic hypotension (dizziness when standing or sitting), fludrocortisone can be used due to its mineralcorticoid and glucocorticoid activity. Also, DHEA can be supportive of the adrenals and has been found to be helpful in autoimmune diseases, insulin resistance, osteoporosis, and atherosclerosis.

The bottom line from all this discussion is that we need to reduce inflammation caused by stress in all its forms. Because even though you can't feel it, your body is inflamed on a molecular level, and it is this "inflammaging" that ages us and makes us sick. The combination of the interventions discussed work synergistically to reduce this oxidative inflammation that will help heal your body from the adrenals up.

It doesn't matter whether the stress in our lives is emotional, nutritional, or environmental: it all affects us - our longevity and our quality-of - life in a negative way. All stress was meant to be temporary. The good stress that helps us optimize our performance has now metastasized into something malignant because of the level of stress we're exposed to.

The dilemma is that there has to be a fine balance of good, performance-enhancing cortisol flowing in your body and a state of relaxation. Finding the correct stress level for you can be compared to playing a violin: if the string is too tight, it's going to break, and if it's too loose, you can't play.

How we cope with stress is dependent on our genetics, our individual coping mechanisms developed early in our lives, our gender, and the type of stressors we are placed under. As well, it is dependent on our ability to participate in leisure activities that dissipate and manage the stress that is found in each of us. How this stress is managed will ultimately impact our longevity and the quality of life we will live. Those who cannot manage their stress will pay a heavy price with chronic disease and disability and an early death.

The good news is that adaptive behavior to manage our stress can be learned, and intervention strategies can be employed that will help prevent and reduce the damage caused by adrenal dysfunction from prolonged stress. Using East and West approaches to medicine, my ultimate goal for my patients – and all people – is to help them achieve an active and healthy quality of life so they can enjoy their lives fully and fulfill the life span that was granted to them.

Dr. Roger Garcia

Dr. Roger Garcia has devoted his practice to preventative medicine and believes that humankind was meant to enjoy the blessing of a long life.

Dr. Garcia earned his medical degree from the Ohio University College of Osteopathic Medicine (1983). He also holds a law degree from Capital University Law School (1996) and was "of counsel" for a prominent Columbus, Ohio, law firm for a number of years. He has served as director of The Bellevue Hospital's emergency department, where he is also an Assistant Professor of Emergency Medicine.

Dr. Garcia is the author of *Aged to Perfection: Anti-aging, Wellness & Weight Loss with Natural Bioidentical Hormones*, which discusses how to live a full life through good nutrition, fitness, stress reduction, and hormonal balance using bioidentical hormone therapy.

His interest in age-related health issues led to board certification and a fellowship in functional and regenerative medicine from the American Academy of Anti-Aging Medicine. He also has certifications in family and emergency medicine and is a certified independent medical examiner.

The father of six-year-old twin daughters, Dr. Garcia lives his beliefs in a vigorous lifestyle, which includes adventures such as running with the bulls in Spain.

Dr. Roger Garcia
Suite 100, 1120 Polaris Parkway
Columbus, Ohio, United States
43240

Phone: 877-501-4287
E-mail: rgarrcia@yahoo.com
www.perfectedwellness.com

CHAPTER FIVE

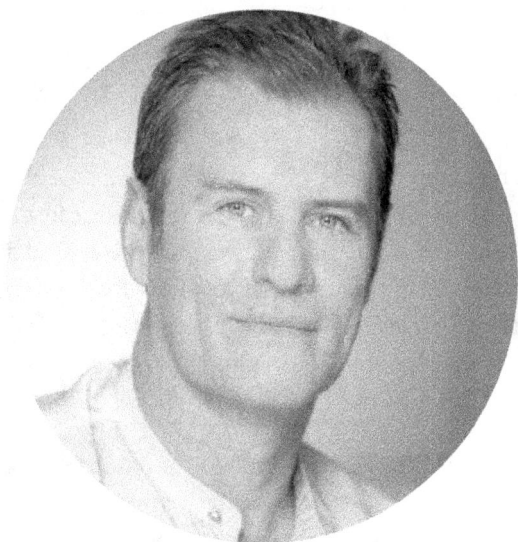

Dr. Bruce Hoffman:

Male Menopause

CHAPTER FIVE

Dr. Bruce Hoffman: Male Menopause

I f you've read about "male menopause," you probably know about testosterone. Dropping levels of testosterone cause many of the complaints, such as the mid-life crisis of the typical grumpy man. If the hormones in the body work together like the members of a band, testosterone plays lead guitar, while estrogen is on vocals. If the testosterone level fades, estrogen begins to overpower, and, before long, the whole band plays out of tune.

So a better overall balance of hormones is required as a man grows older. The thing is, this involves not only testosterone and estrogen, but also all the other hormones. The challenge is noticing the discord when it starts, because the first few bad notes may be subtle and are often blamed on stress or simply getting older.

Sound Check

Men don't usually come to the doctor's office complaining about male menopause, also called andropause. The more common scenario is a fifty-something executive, slightly overweight, appearing exhausted and irritable, reluctantly arriving for a check-up. This usually doesn't occur until his wife, asking about her menopausal status the week before, mentions to the doctor, "You know, I think my husband should come and see you. He hasn't been himself lately. He's grumpy. He lies down on the couch any chance he can get. He complains of vague aches and pains and I can't remember the last time we had sex!"

By asking a few probing questions, the doctor finds out that the man's symptoms were slower and more insidious in onset than his wife's but, nevertheless, just as dramatic in their outcome. Men traditionally tend to have a more stoic and fatalistic approach to encroaching signs and symptoms, but as an imbalance in hormone levels typically affects a man's sexual performance first, this is often what propels him to seek medical attention.

The danger of ignoring all the other signs of declining hormone levels – those off-key notes of the band – is that andropause is not necessarily a harmless, "natural" process. It often comes with major physical and mental changes that, over the long term, can have a dramatic effect on slowly developing diseases.

But exactly what do these changes involve, and when do they start?

Highs and Lows

Male menopause is a gradual shift in hormonal, physiological, and chemical balances that occurs in all men between the ages of forty and fifty-five, although it can occur as early as thirty-five and as late as sixty-five. Incidentally, the term "hormone," is derived from the Greek word hormo, which means to set in motion. This is precisely what hormones do.

Hormones are involved in almost every biological process, including sexual reproduction, growth, metabolism, and your body's immune response. It's no wonder that the symptoms of andropause are so varied and widespread. Hormones stimulate, regulate, and control the function of various tissues and organs and are manufactured by specialized groups of cells in your glands. These glands—which include the hypothalamus, pituitary, thyroid, adrenals, ovaries, and testes—

release the hormones into the body as they're needed.

The Slow Fall

The following hormone levels decline as a man ages:

- Testosterone
- Growth hormone
- Melatonin
- Dehydroepiandrosterone (DHEA)
- Progesterone
- Pregnenolone
- Oxytocin

The Gradual Rise

The following hormone levels go up with andropause:

- Estrogen
- Insulin
- Cortisol

As mentioned before, testosterone is the lead guitarist in the aging man's band of hormones – when it begins to fade, estrogen takes over, with detrimental effects.

Why Low Levels of Testosterone are Dangerous

Studies have shown that too little testosterone in the aging man's blood is linked to the following:

- Heart disease
- Declining memory
- Anxiety
- Depression
- Alzheimer's disease
- Diabetes and metabolic syndrome
- Loss of muscle mass and strength

- Loss of bone thickness and strength
- A greater chance of dying from any cause

The fears around testosterone replacement therapy and whether it may cause prostate cancer have also been laid to rest by definitive studies. But what about the effects of all the other fading players in the hormone band?

DHEA

DHEA is a hormone made by the adrenal glands, gonads (testicles and ovaries), brain, and skin in both men and women. It also declines with advancing age. By the time we are seventy to eighty years of age, peak levels of DHEA are only 10-20 percent of those in young adults.

As DHEA is the most important and abundant steroid hormone and the precursor of all other sex hormones, it serves extremely well to help restore many functions in the body. Low levels of DHEA are associated with aging and most diseases of aging.

Studies have shown that the dramatic age-related drop in DHEA levels is accompanied by an equally dramatic rise in heart disease. It seems DHEA is incorporated into both HDL ("good" cholesterol) and LDL ("bad" cholesterol) and helps to protect both from becoming oxidized – a process that spells trouble for the heart and arteries. As our DHEA levels drop with age, less of this hormone is available to protect our cholesterol, and the more at risk we are of developing heart problems.

It's well known that cortisol, the stress hormone, harms the brain. But DHEA, due to its action in keeping cortisol in check, appears to protect the brain from these damaging effects.

Many of the diseases of aging—such as heart disease, Alzheimer's, certain cancers, diabetes, and osteoporosis—are linked in one way or another to inflammation. Studies have shown that DHEA is an effective anti-inflammatory, and the ability to maintain youthful levels of this hormone as we age may play a key role in protecting us from these inflammatory diseases.

DHEA is also a mood modulator. One study showed that supplementing with 50mg of DHEA every night for six months in both men and women, aged forty to seventy, improved energy levels, quality of sleep, mood, and the ability to handle stress.

Consider doing the following to boost your DHEA levels naturally:

- Eat a low-calorie diet containing less than 40g of carbohydrates per day.
- Exercise and meditate.
- Take part in creative, physical activities that reduce stress.

Growth Hormone

A drop in growth hormone (GH) as you grow older can also have a dramatic effect on your sense of well-being. GH has multiple protective roles and is responsible for the body's major growth spurt during puberty. In adulthood, GH maintains skin, muscle, and bone health. With a deficiency of this hormone, signs of aging are quickly accelerated. Skin wrinkles and sags; fat soon replaces muscle.

Growth hormone also helps maintain and repair the health of various organs, including the heart, lungs, liver, kidneys, joints, nerves, and brain. As growth hormone activates the calming, regenerative parasympathetic nervous system, a deficiency may result in increased tension, anxiety, and depression and a decreased ability to cope with stress.

From the age of thirty onward, growth hormone levels decline fairly rapidly, about 1-3 percent per year. This loss is quickly accelerated if you're obese. The most efficient way to replace growth hormone is through a daily injection, similar to a diabetic insulin shot.

Most anti-aging doctors will not treat GH in the first year of restoring optimal hormone levels, as a protein-rich diet; an adequate sleep and exercise program; and the replacement of testosterone, progesterone, melatonin, and thyroid levels may increase GH levels by as much as 20-30 percent.. Treatment with growth hormone begins only when all the other hormone levels in the body have been brought back to normal.

Consider doing the following to boost your GH levels naturally:

- Supplement your diet with amino acids.
- Exercise daily.
- Make sure all the other hormones are at youthful levels.
- Eat a diet rich in proteins.
- Avoid alcohol, sugar, sweets, breads, and pasta.
- Lose weight.
- Avoid milk products.
- Avoid sleep deprivation.
- Avoid prolonged stress.

Progesterone

Men typically produce between 1.5-3mg of progesterone per day. But as men age, their progesterone levels fall exponentially.

Progesterone is used in the production of cortisol, the stress hormone. So if a man leads a particularly stressful life, it's very likely he will have low levels of progesterone. Progesterone is vital in keeping the higher levels of estrogen in aging men in check and thus minimizing the risk of heart attacks, prostate enlargement, and prostate cancer. A typical dose of progesterone may lower estradiol levels – a cancer-causing form of estrogen – by up to 30 percent. Progesterone also lowers the hormone responsible for causing hair loss and baldness in men, called dihydrotestosterone (DHT), while reducing water retention and possibly high blood pressure.

Consider doing the following to boost your progesterone levels naturally:

- Eat a diet rich in protein.
- Manage stress daily with stress-reduction techniques.
- Use herbs and supplements such as Rhodiola rosea, Siberian ginseng, licorice root extract, ashwaganda and vitamins B5 and C.

Melatonin

Melatonin, the sleep hormone, is another hormone to keep an eye on with advancing age.

Melatonin has a positive effect on the part of our nervous system involved in rest and relaxation. In particular, melatonin plays a part in slowing the release of adrenalin, so without enough of it, the body reacts with a fight-or-flight response. Melatonin may also improve your sexual performance, particularly enhancing serenity and relaxation after sex.

Signs that you may be deficient include light, restless sleep with many anxious thoughts; easy waking during the night; difficulty falling asleep and falling back asleep once you're awake; poor dreaming or dream recall; anxiety at night; depression (especially the winter blues); excessive emotionality and irritability; and restless leg syndrome with increased muscle spasms. You may also have intestinal spasms or cramps.

Studies have linked a melatonin deficiency to hypertension, artery disease, heartbeat irregularity, obesity, diabetes, osteoporosis, lowered immunity with recurrent infections, breast and prostate cancer, and brain diseases like Parkinson's and Alzheimer's disease.

Melatonin supplements should be taken at bedtime, either under the tongue or in pill form. They work best when you combine them with Vitamin B6 and tryptophan or 5-hydroxytryptophan, which convert to melatonin with the help of Vitamin B6. Some asthmatics may react negatively to melatonin, so use with care if you're an asthma sufferer.

Consider doing the following to boost your melatonin levels naturally:

- Increase your exposure to morning daylight (use a sunlamp if needed).
- Make the room pitch-black at night or use an eye mask.
- Avoid alcohol and caffeinated drinks.
- Avoid stressful activities.
- Avoid electromagnetic exposure at night such as from cell phones or electrical clocks and radios.
- Wear turquoise-colored glasses thirty minutes before bed.

Pregnenolone

Pregnenolone is made from cholesterol and is the mother of many hormones, including DHEA, testosterone, estradiol, progesterone, cortisol, and aldosterone. In addition to functioning as a hormone, it also serves as a brain chemical, or neurotransmitter, in specific areas of the brain responsible for memory. Pregnenolone regulates the flow of calcium through the cell membrane, and this process determines how memory is encoded by our nerve cells.

In addition, pregnenolone increases the levels of the neurotransmitter acetylcholine, the brain chemical responsible for creating memories as well as assisting the main part of the brain that stores memory. The most common complaints of men with pregnenolone deficiency include memory loss and joint pain as well as dry skin and fatigue. Replacement doses are typically 30mg twice a day for memory loss.

You may choose to use other brain-boosting foods and supplements such as the following:

- Acetyl-L-carnitine
- Vinpocetine
- Phosphatidyl serine, combined with omega-3 fatty acids
- Phosphatidylcholine
- DMAE

- G6PC
- Huperizine
- Vitamin D
- Blueberries

Oxytocin

Oxytocin, a hormone known to improve social bonding, is made by the pituitary gland in the brain. It helps us fall in love, spurs parenting instincts, and intensifies orgasms.

Studies have found that similar to women, men report an improved sexual response when using an oxytocin nasal spray, including stronger feelings of tenderness and closeness with the sexual partner before, during, and after sex.

The following aspects boost oxytocin levels naturally:
- Romantic love
- Hugging
- Soft touching
- Massage
- Orgasm
- Partner support
- Singing
- Physical exercise
- Warm climate
- Positive environment
- Reading
- Positive social contacts
- Viewing pictures of loved ones
- Living with others

Armed with information about the importance of youthful hormone levels, men have no reason not to stay completely tuned in to the music of life, no matter their age.

FELICIA PIZZONIA, R.H.N

Dr. Bruce Hoffman

Dr. Bruce Hoffman, an impassioned doctor and healer, is a key contributor to the revolution in conventional medicine. He earned his medical degree from the University of Cape Town, South Africa, in 1981. In 1985, he moved to Canada, and he is now Medical Director of The Hoffman Centre for Integrative Medicine in Calgary, Alberta, (www.hoffmancentre.com) and consults in both countries.

In the early 1990s, Dr. Hoffman realized the limitations of his traditional medical training and began an extensive study of the disciplines of integrative medicine. He has studied anti-aging medicine and bioidentical hormone replacement therapy, chelation, IV nutrient therapy, neural and prolotherapy, hellerwork, homotoxicology, energy psychology, ayurvedic medicine, traditional Chinese medicine, family constellation therapy, and the Demartini method, among others. He has also trained with leading mind-body and spiritual healers such as Deepak Chopra and Dr. John Demartini.

Dr. Hoffman received board certification in anti-aging and regenerative medicine in 2008 and received his fellowship qualification from the American Academy of Anti-Aging Medicine in 2009. Presently, he's completing a master's degree in nutrition and metabolic medicine from the University of South Florida.

His unified model of healing, called the "7 Stages to Health and Transformation™," provides an inspiring vision of detoxification, healing, and self-actualization. The DVD and workbook is currently available, and a book is to be published by the end of the year.

Dr. Bruce Hoffman
The Hoffman Centre for Integrative Medicine
1133 17th Avenue NW
Calgary, Alberta, Canada
T2M 0P7

Phone: 403-206-2333 (Reception Ext. 201)
www. hoffmancentre.com
E-mail: info@hoffmancentre.com

CHAPTER SIX

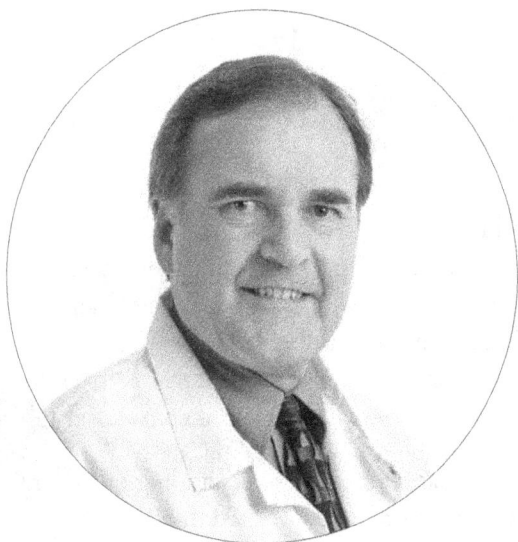

Dr. Randall LaFrom:

The Oral-Systemic Connection

CHAPTER SIX

Dr. Randall LaFrom:
The Oral-Systemic Connection

According to recent reports from both the Mayo Clinic and from Dr. Mehmet Oz, flossing your teeth can add six to ten years to your life. Who wouldn't want to do that? The problem is that flossing alone does not address the deeper issues of oral inflammation or the presence of cavity-forming bacteria in our saliva. This is why a larger view of oral health is so necessary.

Newer technology and a better understanding of the oral-systemic, or mouth-body, connection have advanced the modern dentist's role from "just" restoring cavities and missing teeth and identifying bleeding gums to one that connects your oral problems with your general health. These "oral physicians" play a critical role in a patient's overall well-being and are as important as any of the other medical specialists.

In this chapter, you will learn not only how your overall dental health can affect your body, but also how your overall health can be reflected by the conditions in your mouth.

It's well recognized that a poorly maintained oral cavity opens passages for toxins and bacteria into the circulatory system, most often from bleeding gums. Also, additional risk factors such as lifestyle, nutrition, drugs, and undiagnosed diseases can manifest symptoms in your mouth. It is therefore critical that a dentist conducts a comprehensive medical history for all his patients before treatment.

With the proliferation of popular medications that have dry mouth as an undesired side effect, more people have acidic saliva, which has become a leading cause of severe tooth decay. This is exacerbated by external factors, including the following:

- Frequent consumption of acidic beverages (sodas, coffee, wine)
- Frequent consumption of sugar-laden snacks and carbohydrates
- Gastric reflux (when acidic stomach liquids back up into the esophagus)
- Bulimia (eating disorder characterized by binge eating often followed by vomiting, fasting, or taking of laxatives)
- Smoking and drug and alcohol use

Dentists have become detectives in assessing risks and trying to identify the underlying causes of tooth decay and other oral conditions so that successful treatment plans can be developed. Fortunately, modern dentists now have the tools to conduct comprehensive oral exams. Most critical exams include those for temporomandibular joint (TMJ) disorder, tissue lesions or ulcers, oral cancer, bleeding gums, tooth mobility, bone loss, cavities, fractured teeth and fillings, overly worn or misaligned teeth, plaque, and sleep apnea. In addition, many new diagnostic tests are available now that allow simple and non-invasive assessment of saliva flow and pH as well as risk factors for various diseases, including diabetes, certain cancers, and Alzheimer's.

Two primary factors that contribute to the aging or deterioration in the body are pH imbalance and inflammation. These manifest themselves in the mouth as cavities and gum disease. In the next two sections, I will address each of these concepts in more detail.

Salivary Diagnostics and pH

The role of saliva in maintaining optimal dental health is often underestimated. Saliva offers enzymes and proteins to help break down and lubricate food, making it easier to swallow, and provides anti-microbial activity for teeth. It also helps neutralize acidic foods and drinks that contact your teeth, protecting them. It's important to realize that in an acidic environment, teeth start to slowly dissolve on the surface, allowing bacteria to enter and form cavities. Therefore, a more pH-neutral environment with a normal saliva flow rate is desired for a healthy mouth.

Tests identifying saliva quantity and pH and potential genetic markers for certain health conditions are some of the tools for a patient's overall health risk assessment. Your salivary conditions have a significant impact on your oral and systemic health.

If a person has "dry mouth" (xerostomia), the saliva's critical acid balance can get offset from mouth breathing, radiation therapy, smoking, or one of hundreds of prescription medications (high blood pressure, diuretics, asthma, antihistamines, allergy, anti-depressants, anti-anxiety, sleeping and pain pills, anti-inflammatories, and decongestants, to name a few). The resulting lower saliva flow and pH drop creates a huge increase in the risk of cavities.

Health conditions such as diabetes, Sjogren's syndrome, HIV/AIDS, Parkinson's disease, high blood pressure, snoring, GERD, nerve damage, and cancer can all contribute to dry mouth and/or low pH.

When a patient with a long history of healthy teeth suddenly has multiple cavities, it's important for the dentist to investigate what medications, health conditions, lifestyle changes, habits, or new therapies have occurred in that patient's life. Often, I may find a patient who has started on a new medication that dries out his or her mouth. These patients will often start sucking on candies, breath mints, or lozenges - many with a high sugar content - to increase saliva flow, without even realizing that there's an underlying problem developing. Many physicians may not be as familiar with the consequences of a dry mouth.

Saliva provides a protective layer on teeth that contains calcium, phosphate, and proteins that regulate the intake and loss of minerals on the tooth's surface. While no single species of bacteria is identified as the cause of cavities, Streptococcus mutans is frequently found in higher amounts in those with more cavities. Cavities typically develop in areas where the microbial deposits sit on the teeth and form a biofilm. The bacteria, when exposed to sugars, create a layer of plaque on the teeth and, if left undisturbed, can lead to decay.

The bacteria that thrive in acidic environments also produce acid from the sugars and contribute to demineralization of the teeth. This most commonly occurs in the deep grooves on the top of the teeth, deeper in between teeth near the roots, or under defective margins on fillings or crowns. Simply drilling and filling the holes will not stop the problem, since a cavity is the manifestation of a bacterial infection.

Some liquids, such as soda, often contain phosphoric acid, which is especially damaging to the teeth. Alcohol, coffee, tea, and sports drinks often have a low pH as well and, if left on the teeth for prolonged periods, can also damage them. The pH of these drinks is below the pH at which calcium is depleted from the tooth. Note that brushing immediately after drinking these is also not recommended, as it is like brushing your teeth with acid! Instead, rinse with water or chew a sugar-free gum, wait a short time, and/or use an acid-neutralizing toothpaste to cleanse the teeth.

The salivary pH ideally should be at or above seven, but throughout the day, especially after a meal, the pH may drop into the decay zone (high to severe acidity, pH below 5.5). The root surfaces of the teeth and the areas around the edge of restorations begin to wash out at a pH below 6.4.

For most people, salivary pH will rise back into their normal range within one hour after eating. Dry-mouth patients, however, do not have the saliva flow to buffer or flush away the acids and often need additional, specialized oral hygiene habits, products, and/or therapies. Studies from the Centers for Disease Control and Prevention indicate that in some populations, as high as 92 percent of adults have had cavities. When left untreated, cavities often lead to tooth loss and infection. This indicates that the public is not being properly educated on the causes and prevention of cavities.

Salivary pH can be determined easily by a simple litmus paper test. A patient's goal is to keep the pH above the demineralization range for the longest amount of time each day to have the least amount of decay. By reducing the intake of acidic drinks and sugary foods, removing or modifying the biofilm on the teeth through proper home care and professional cleanings, and maintaining the oral saliva pH between 6.8-7.2, the risk of developing cavities can be significantly reduced.

Patients with pH challenges should consider increasing water intake, using a baking soda toothpaste, or using xylitol-containing products (gums, mints, lozenges, candies, or rinses) that have been shown to have antibacterial properties and reduce tooth demineralization.

Sustained pH therapy is especially important for patients on long-term medications or with conditions such as diabetes or cancer, who also typically suffer from low salivary pH. As dentists, we tend to find that diabetics are at significantly higher risk not only for decay, but also for bone loss and bleeding gums. Keeping their oral pH in the 6.6-7.0 or higher (alkaline) range for long periods of time can minimize the deterioration. Ask your dentist for a home pH-testing kit.

In our practice, when reviewing ten-year histories of patients' dental care, we found that patients who had a consistent pH of below 6.2 needed nearly four times the amount of dental treatment (measured in dollars) compared to those with 6.8 or above. When comparing patients with 5.8 pH and below to those with 7.0 and above, the difference jumped to six times the amount of care.

Not only were we seeing that patients with the consistently low salivary pH were having significantly higher cavity rates, but they also needed more root canals, crowns, and extractions. This included a 300 percent higher number of repeat cavities on the same teeth over the ten-year period. These findings were consistent with those of Dr. V. Kim Kutsch of Oral BioTech, who conducted independent studies showing that prolonged periods of low oral pH played a more significant role in cavities than did genetics, quantity of sugar eaten, or specific bacteria.

From a nutritional point of view, when patients switch to higher alkaline foods, typically vegetables, and eat less acidic foods such as meats and carbohydrates (like bread and cakes), they can raise their oral pH. Drinking more water and consuming less soda, coffee, tea, and alcohol can also help raise pH. Many studies show that increasing consumption of broccoli and cheese assists with providing calcium and phosphorus, which provide nutrients for enamel remineralization. Eating seeds and nuts have also been shown to inhibit the onset of cavities.

A full discussion on nutrition is beyond the scope of this article. While we know that some foods provide useful nutrients, the quantities, ratios of nutrients in the foods, and the concerns for allergies can be argued and discussed through forums and in books or articles found online. Suffice it to say that improper nutrition does play a significant role in the development of cavities and gum disease.

Periodontal Disease

The second thing that affects aging and health is inflammation. It is the body's response to infection and irritation. One of the most common chronic infections in adults is periodontitis (gum disease).

Periodontitis, an inflammation of the tissues surrounding the teeth, is caused by bacteria and can result in progressive loss of gum tissue and the jawbone supporting the teeth. It is the most common cause of tooth loss. Tooth loss not only affects confidence, aesthetics, and speech, but also the ability to chew food, which can cause digestive problems.

Infectious periodontitis has been shown to increase the body's inflammatory response and has been associated with an increase in cardiovascular diseases, including strokes and atherosclerosis. Numerous studies have shown that periodontitis should be included with other risk factors for evaluating a patient's chances for cardiovascular disease.

The body's inflammatory response from gum disease leads to an increase in messenger molecules that cause the liver to produce and release C-reactive proteins (CRPs) into the blood. Trauma, cancer, stress, smoking, and poor diet can also cause a rise in CRPs. A simple test of high sensitivity CRP in the blood can determine a patient's risk level for cardiovascular disease even more accurately than high levels of LDL cholesterol.

One of the modifiable risk factors for periodontal disease is smoking. The heat from a cigarette can diminish the blood supply, limiting the ability of nutrients and oxygen to get to the tissues. Secondly, the chemicals in smoke suppress the body's defense mechanism, compromising the immune system and making smokers (especially if diabetic) more susceptible to infection that might contribute to periodontal disease.

Airborne diseases like tuberculosis, pneumonia, influenza, scarlet fever, measles, and rheumatic fever are known to attack the body through the oral cavity. It is now recognized that inflamed and bleeding periodontal pockets can easily pass oral bacteria directly into the bloodstream. Those bacteria can be associated with cardiovascular diseases, diabetes, and arthritis. Women with periodontitis are at seven times higher risk for pre-term, low birthweight delivery.

In almost all cases, gum inflammation is caused by bacteria from infection or aggravation from plaque. Theoretically, proper and diligent oral hygiene, including brushing and flossing, is capable of preventing these conditions by reducing the amount of food, disease-causing bacteria, and biofilm built up on teeth. Periodontitis is a complex disease, with common signs and symptoms, but they don't all have to be present for the disease to be active. For this reason, treatment or prevention of periodontal disease is not straightforward.

In most cases, simple mechanical scaling and root planing will help minimize the symptoms, but it is not enough on its own to get rid of periodontal disease. Often, nutritional counseling to help improve the body's defense mechanisms along with antibiotics and modifications in home care are suggested to address the disease. In some cases, bacterial cultures are needed to determine the presence of specific bacteria. Through the use of specific antibiotics, we can destroy these organisms. When antibiotics are taken orally, the entire body is affected. In rare cases, systemic use of antibiotics can lead to undesired side effects or even an increased risk of developing resistant bacterial strains or fungal infections. Whenever possible, medications should be delivered locally to avoid systemic side effects.

Newer techniques involve giving lower dosages of antibiotics that are not designed to kill the bacteria but to regulate the body's own immune response to manage inflammation. These new antibiotic techniques are especially welcome for people with physical disabilities, who may lack the manual dexterity to practice good oral hygiene. Patients with Parkinson's, cerebral palsy, autism, or even Down syndrome can have more than a 90 percent higher risk for periodontal disease. Sustained-release lozenges that deliver bacteria-killing ingredients, impede biofilm formation and plaque buildup, and elevate saliva pH into the neutral range are products used in the prevention of dental decay, gingivitis, and periodontitis.

Snoring and Sleep Apnea

Snoring is often a symptom of a breathing obstruction while sleeping. Losing weight, avoiding alcohol, or sleeping on your side can help limit snoring. Snoring may be one of the symptoms of a more potentially dangerous condition called obstructive sleep apnea (OSA). As much as 80 percent of those people who involuntarily grind or clench their teeth may have some degree of OSA.

OSA screening can be done by a dentist in a routine check-up. Diagnosis is based on the Epworth sleepiness scale, a questionnaire discussing eight situations where a person might doze off. Once OSA is proven, it's important to conduct overnight sleep studies using more sensitive tools such as polysomnography, which records internal biological changes that occur during sleep.

Sleep apnea can be the result of multiple areas of airway collapse in the head and neck, including the tongue, jaws, chin, soft palate, tonsils, epiglottis, and pharyngeal walls. In many cases, a bite splint that repositions and moves the lower jaw forward may be enough to open the airway. There are levels of apnea, some of which can be treated with a continuous positive airway pressure machine. In more advanced OSA cases, surgical correction may be required.

Lack of treatment for sleep apnea can lead to stress, drowsiness, headaches, dry mouth, personality changes, or other complications, including increased risk of stroke and cardiovascular problems. In addition, there is a higher risk of sleep apnea in patients who have gastric reflux. Complications from apnea can contribute to both dental and overall health risks.

The Oral-systemic Link

Hopefully, this article has shown how systemic diseases can affect the mouth as well as how the mouth can reflect what's happening with the rest of the body.

In the United States today, diabetes currently affects 10 percent of the adult population. The Centers for Disease Control claims that with current trends in the known risk factors we are observing, that number could climb to as much as one-third of the U.S. adult population by the year 2050. Since diabetes has been shown to result in more common mouth ulcers, cavities, dry mouth, tooth loss, and bone loss, it's one of the most critical and growing areas of research in oral-systemic healthcare. In addition, gum disease worsens diabetes. It's a vicious cycle. A person can reduce their risk of diabetes by about 50 percent just by following the CDC's guidelines.

Studies released in 2010 by the American Academy of Periodontology showed that the incidence of periodontal disease was previously underestimated and that as much as 90 percent of adults over age fifty have some form of periodontal disease. Since the connection between periodontal disease and cardiovascular disease has been well established, this should be a priority in patients' conversations with their dentists and doctors.

It's well established that to live a healthy life, your mouth has to be healthy, too. It's important to involve a patient's general physician if and when any potential medical complication or medical interactions have been identified.

The next time you visit your dentist or physician, be sure to notify them of all the things that are going on with you and the medications you are taking and symptoms you are experiencing. Tell your dentist if you have had bleeding gums, dry mouth, ulcers that don't heal, frequent thirst, or loose teeth. If you are female, let them know if you are pregnant or thinking about becoming pregnant. Let your medical doctor know if you have been diagnosed with periodontal disease or are experiencing dry mouth.

When selecting a dentist, consider looking for an oral physician who understands the interactions of the oral-systemic connection. Your doctor should spend time teaching you how to prevent and avoid dental treatment with a thorough review of risk factors, including pH and saliva testing and a review of medications, medical conditions, nutrition, and finally, proper oral hygiene. By choosing a knowledgeable oral physician, you can make sure your dentist's "Open wide!" is followed by an "All clear!" for your long-term health.

Further information and references for sources for this article can be found at www.TheOralPhysician.com.

Further information about oral systemic health can be found at the American Academy for Oral Systemic Health website or on my personal website: www.AAOSH.com, www.LaFrom.com.

Dr. Randall LaFrom

Dr. Randall LaFrom maintains a private practice in Santa Clara County, California. "Dr. Randy" knew he wanted to be a dentist since the fourth grade. He has remained committed to his passion of making sure his patients have the best, state-of-the-art treatment possible in a caring environment.

Dr. LaFrom loves being a continuous student, attending every seminar and sharing what he learns with others. He lives by this quote from Barbara Viniar, who says, "It is essential that along with imparting facts, that we inspire the ability and desire to learn."

After attending San Jose State University, Dr. LaFrom graduated from UCLA Dental School in 1982. He's been serving the Silicon Valley community for more than twenty-seven years in his practice, Advanced Technology Dental Care Center of Cupertino. He's a member of the American Dental Association, California Dental Association, Santa Clara County Dental Society, American Academy of Cosmetic Dentistry, and the World Congress of Minimally Invasive Dentistry and is a founding member of the newly formed American Academy for Oral Systemic Health.

Dr. LaFrom is a contributing healthcare expert author on several websites including:

www.TheOralPhysician.com,
www.wellsphere.com and
www.buzymoms.com

His office website is www.LaFrom.com.

Randall LaFrom, DDS
Advanced Technology Dental Care Center of Cupertino
COSMETIC AND GENERAL DENTISTRY
Suite B, 20445 Pacifica Drive
Cupertino, California, United States
95014

Phone: 408-996-8595
E-mail: drlafrom@yahoo.com
www.lafrom.com

CHAPTER SEVEN

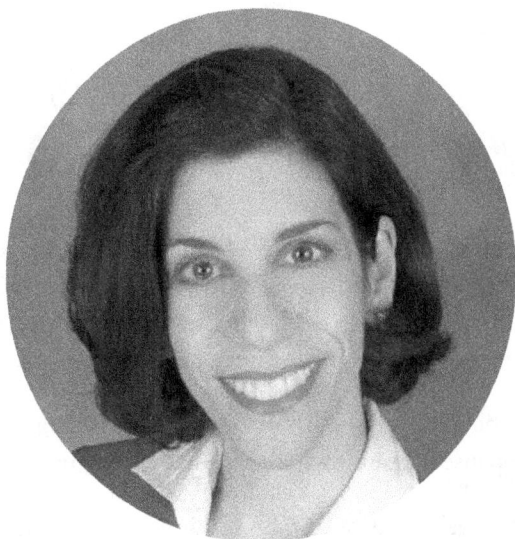

Dr. Susan Linder:

Pellet Therapy

CHAPTER SEVEN

Dr. Susan Linder: Pellet Therapy

Within our bodies, we contain a symphony of hormones.

Hormones are chemicals that send messages from the cells in one part of the body to cells in another. These hormones are vital; they control everything from our growth, to sex drive, metabolism, the strength of our bones, and memory.

As you age, the body releases fewer hormones, leading to conditions such as menopause and andropause, also known as "male menopause."

My goal as a physician is to get all of those hormones in harmony so you can be the best, healthiest you – the version of you that nature intended.

One aspect of hormone replacement therapy that I've personally seen to be extraordinarily effective in helping my patients is pellet therapy. What is pellet therapy? The pellet is a way of delivering so-called "bioidentical" hormones, which are often derived from plants and made to match those that exist in the human body naturally. I feel that using these bioidentical hormones is best, because they work like a lock and key. When the proper key (hormone) is found, it will make the lock (cell receptor) work properly, and the right signal will come through to the cell.

Pellets were frequently used in the United States from about 1940 through the late 1970s when oral patented estrogens were marketed to the public. Today, pellets are used here as well as frequently in Europe and Australia. I have implanted well over one thousand pellets in hundreds of patients and have seen very positive responses.

When compared to conventional hormones in clinical studies, pellets have been shown to be superior for relief of menopausal symptoms, maintenance of bone density, restoration of sleep patterns, and improvement in sex drive, libido, and sexual response and performance. In women, testosterone pellets help with vaginal dryness, incontinence, and urinary urgency and frequency. In both men and women, testosterone has been shown to increase energy and sense of well-being, relieve depression and anxiety, and improve memory and concentration. Testosterone pellets may be used in pre-menopausal females (women who have not stopped menstruating). Testosterone has been shown to relieve migraine or menstrual headaches, help with symptoms of PMS (pre-menstrual syndrome), relieve anxiety and depression, increase energy, help with sleep, and improve sex drive and libido. If a pre-menopausal female has a testosterone pellet inserted, she must use birth control. There is a theoretical risk of 'masculinizing' a female fetus (giving male traits to a female fetus).

Testosterone delivered by pellet implant increases lean body mass (muscle strength, bone density) and decreases fat mass. Both men and women need adequate testosterone levels for optimal mental and physical health and for the prevention of chronic illnesses like Alzheimer's and Parkinson's disease, which are associated with low testosterone levels. Testosterone delivered by pellet implantation has been shown to decrease breast proliferation and lower the risk of breast cancer, even in patients on conventional hormone replacement therapy. Clinical studies show that testosterone balances estrogen and is breast protective. Hormone deficiency is a common cause of hair loss, and treatment with estradiol and testosterone implants can help to re-grow hair. Hair becomes thicker and less dry with pellet therapy.

Most men maintain adequate levels of testosterone into their mid-forties to mid-fifties. Men should be tested when they begin to show signs of testosterone deficiency. Even men in their thirties can be testosterone deficient and show signs of bone loss, fatigue, depression, erectile dysfunction, difficulty sleeping, and mental decline. Most men need to be tested around fifty years of age. It is never too late to benefit from hormone therapy.

Pellets, or implants, are made up of hormones (i.e., testosterone) that are pressed or fused into very small solid cylinders. These pellets are no bigger than a 'Tic Tac' and no smaller than a grain of rice. The pellets are inserted under local anesthesia in the lower abdominal wall or upper buttocks through a small incision, which is then closed with a skin tape (steri-strip). The experience of the physician is very important, not only in placing the pellets, but also in determining the correct dosage of hormones to be used. Pellets deliver a consistent, healthy level of hormones for an average of three to four months in women and five to six months in men. They're embedded under the skin and slowly release whatever hormone you need into your body. They avoid the fluctuations, or ups and downs, of hormone levels seen with other methods of delivery. This is optimal for health and disease prevention. The new hormone level is maintained for the next four to six months, and the pellet does not need to be removed, as it simply dissolves.

Pellets do not increase the risk of blood clots like conventional or synthetic hormone replacement therapy. After pellet implantation, most patients notice improvement in their symptoms within twenty-four to forty-eight hours, while others may take a week or two to notice a difference. Diet and lifestyle, along with hormone balance, are critical for optimal health. Stress is a major contributor to hormone imbalance and illness.

To determine if a person is a candidate for hormone replacement therapy, I always do a thorough patient history, pertinent physical examination, and comprehensive laboratory study to determine the diagnosis and develop a customized treatment plan for that person.

The cost for treatment can range from $230 to $600, depending on the hormone dose and the number of pellets needed. For men, who need larger doses than women, the cost can be more. Pellets need to be inserted, depending on the circumstances and the patient's metabolism, two to four times a year. But when you compare the pellets to the cost of traditional medications, they can be very cost-effective and convenient. Pellet implantation has been consistently proven to be more effective than oral, intramuscular, and topical hormone therapy in regards to bone density, sexual function, mood and cognitive function, urinary and vaginal complaints, breast health, lipid profiles, hormone ratios, and metabolites.

When I first began focusing on anti-aging medicine and pellet therapy in 2006, it was amazing and frustrating to me how many conventional doctors weren't supportive. It was often much easier for the busy practitioner to dismiss the patient than to question his or her beliefs and do the research. It's about a patient making an informed choice. But over the years, I've seen more and more people become aware of what bioidentical hormones do and how effective they are. At this point, I have conventional doctors who refer their spouses and family members to me for the bioidentical hormone replacement, including pellet therapy, because of how well it has been shown to work.

I've had so many men and women in my practice who've had an incredible response to pellet therapy. Let me provide you with an example of one such patient; this gentleman was in his late fifties, and he had a low testosterone level. When we gave him testosterone replacement, with pellets, he came back and was just amazed. His hair, which was gray, started coming back to its natural color. He had also been to a visit with his ophthalmologist to get his glasses adjusted, because he was having problems seeing. But his long-time doctor was surprised to let him know his vision had actually improved and he didn't need glasses to read all the letters on the board. His story was really striking for me, because I was able to see the changes that take place when hormones are replaced.

Apart from aging, there are many other reasons people in today's busy and hectic world are suffering from hormone-deficient conditions such as menopause, andropause, adrenal fatigue, and thyroid problems. We're exposed to numerous toxins on a daily basis. They begin in the morning, when women put all these different chemicals on the outside of their bodies: perfumes, shampoos, conditioners, moisturizers, and makeup. And on the inside, we're also eating food that has been genetically modified and contains chemicals and even hormones. We're seeing a lot of toxins in our lives from an environmental standpoint.

If you want to try using food to help increase your hormones, what you need to look at is having a very clean diet. There's no magical food or supplement to increase your body's hormone production: You need to make lifestyle changes and to eat more whole, nutritious foods that haven't been processed and don't contain lots of chemicals. Choose foods with powerful antioxidant properties.

Antioxidants are substances that attack the free radicals moving around in your body that can damage cells and DNA, according to the University of Maryland. Free radicals are naturally occurring, but environmental toxins can increase them. Scientists, according to the University of Maryland, believe that these free radicals can speed up the aging process and lead to heart disease and even cancer. Antioxidants can reduce or prevent such cellular damage.

All of my patients are advised to eat a wide variety of fresh fruits and vegetables, including blueberries, which have a very high antioxidant value. Other Spices, such as garlic or turmeric (a member of the ginger family that's often used in curries), can also play a role in good health.

I also believe that adequate sleep (at least seven to eight hours per night) is one of the most important ways to keep your hormones balanced, and it's so commonly overlooked. I see many of my patients who are so busy that they don't think sleep is that important, or they can't sleep because their hormones are imbalanced. When you don't sleep enough, you're not secreting important hormones, such as the growth hormone, and your body isn't getting adequate repair.

One of my favorite quotes is from Mother Theresa, who said, "In this life, we cannot do great things, we can only do small things with great love." That's also a very appropriate metaphor for the work I do with hormone balancing: Although hormones are small molecules, they have a powerful impact on a person's health and quality of life.

Dr. Susan K. Linder, MD

Dr. Susan K. Linder devotes her Fort Worth, Texas, medical practice to anti-aging and functional medicine. She loves helping women and men balance hormones, improve diet, and maintain a physically fit and healthy lifestyle.

Dr. Linder attended medical school at the University of Texas Southwestern Medical Center in Dallas and completed her physical medicine and rehabilitation residency at Baylor College of Medicine in Houston. She is board certified in physical medicine and rehabilitation and subspecialty board certified in pain medicine. She is a Diplomate of the American Board of Anti-Aging, Functional, and Regenerative Medicine.

Throughout the years that Dr. Linder practiced physical medicine and rehabilitation, she became acutely aware of the devastation caused by sedentary living, a lack of nutrition and fitness, and imbalanced hormones. This discovery motivated her to expand her practice's focus from rehab, physical therapy, and sports medicine to include preventive medicine and bioidentical hormone therapy for men and women. She's an active member of the American Academy of Anti-Aging Medicine and a graduate of the Fellowship in Anti-Aging and Functional Medicine.

Dr. Linder was named a "Health Care Hero" by the Fort Worth Business Press in 2008.

Susan Linder, MD
HealthSpringMD
Suite 203, 2800 S. Hulen
Ft. Worth, Texas, United States
76109

Phone: -817-926-7671
E-mail: info@healthspringmd.com
www.healthspringmd.com

CHAPTER EIGHT

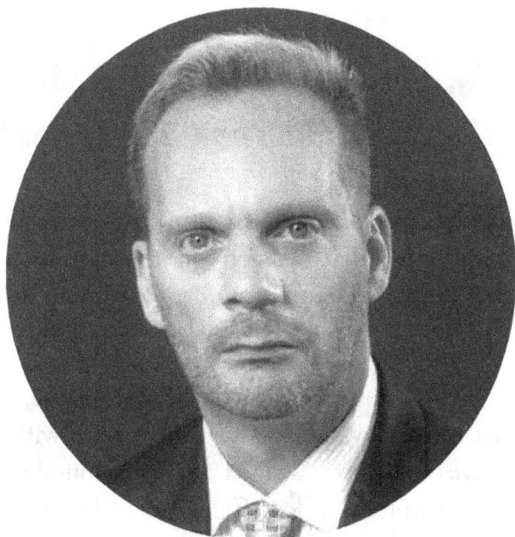

Dr. Paul Savage, MD:
Testosterone Loss and Andropause

CHAPTER EIGHT

Dr. Paul Savage, MD:
Testosterone Loss and Andropause

When people talk about aging, they generally know and understand that women go through menopause, but that's not true for a similar condition in men called andropause.

Andropause, which can also be called male menopause, is the disease specific to men caused by the loss of testosterone with age. But in essence, it involves the physical signs of loss of muscle and strength and the treatable symptoms of loss of energy, vitality, and virility.

Here's a story about me and my own experience with andropause. By the age of thirty-eight, I was not feeling well. I was overweight at 267 pounds, I was stressed, I wasn't sleeping well, my joy for life was gone, and I was depressed.

So I went to see my physician. He told me that I needed to exercise more and eat better. So I did that, religiously. Over a period of six months, however, I didn't lose any weight, and I didn't feel any better. It was my personal trainer who told me, "I think your testosterone is low; you should be on testosterone."

My first instinct was, "Oh my God, no. Testosterone; that's dangerous." Because that's what we're taught. But in thinking about it more, I realized that my trainer probably had a point. I had all the symptoms of low testosterone, including no erections, low libido, depression, inability to gain muscle, inability to lose fat, and low energy level throughout the day.

When I tested my own testosterone level, it came back at around two hundred, which is about the same as an eighty-year-old man. I underwent further testing to make sure that the level wasn't the result of a brain tumor or testicular problem. No, it was simply a low testosterone level. I started treatment with testosterone, and within ten months, I had dropped my body fat from 42 percent down to 20 percent, my muscle mass increased, my energy came up, and the world just came alive. My libido came back, and I was like, "Wow, this stuff is making this total difference in my world." I knew it was the testosterone, because I was already exercising and eating right and wasn't getting the results I needed.

There's a quote I live by: Do a little bit of everything every day. That statement doesn't apply just to hormone replacement. That's a big part of it, but you need proper nutrition, exercise, stress management, sleep, and, if needed, hormone replacement. I always tell my patients that no matter what you do, you have to do a little bit of every one of those everyday activities to be healthy as you age.

What is Testosterone?

Testosterone is a steroid that's made from cholesterol. Anything made from cholesterol is a steroid, and that includes many of the hormones in the body, including Vitamin D, cortisone, testosterone, and estrogen.

Testosterone's function is that of an androgen (a hormone that controls the development and maintenance of male characteristics). It improves a man's mind, mood, muscles, mental processes and mobility. It acts on his body as a builder and an energizer.

When you look at hormones, you're looking at the harmony of all sorts of different hormones that interact and work with each other. So when we're talking about hormonal balance, what we're really talking about is getting the levels of hormones to such a degree that they're actually able to function and interact properly. There's a relationship between testosterone and cortisone hormones. There's a relationship between testosterone and estrogen, the female hormone. There's a relationship between testosterone and insulin, which helps you metabolize your glucose (blood sugar). And most importantly, there are relationships between all hormones.

Increased Recognition

There are multiple reasons that andropause is becoming more prevalent and more discussed.

The primary reason is the recognition of low testosterone as a disease process. We know that it causes increased mortality. Men who have the lowest level of testosterone have the highest rate of mortality, cardiovascular problems, and cancer. So part of the dawning of the andropause age has to do with physicians recognizing a previously unrecognized disease state.

Secondly, public awareness has increased greatly about male menopause. From women, who've always been at the forefront of patient-motivated medical research, we've learned so much about menopause and how to treat women with natural hormones that it is just a logical conclusion that we look at men next.

The third thing is that studies have shown that independent of this recognition by physicians of andropause, testosterone levels currently are lower than even what they were ten and twenty years ago. And although the causes are not yet completely defined, there is a substantial amount of evidence to show that there are things that are toxic in our environment that are causing a decrease in the age at which andropause is now occurring.

Misconceptions about Testosterone

First off, testosterone is a steroid, and steroids have been abused and misused, both by physicians and by sports athletes and bodybuilders.

It's developed a bad reputation as being a substance that can be abused. Most medications that we use in current conventional therapy have the potential to be abused. These medications need to be given correctly by a trained physician at the proper physiologic dose to make sure you get the effect you want, without the side effects you don't want, through a controlled doctor-patient relationship.

Negative press has caused the general public to think, "Testosterone is bad, because it can be abused." But testosterone and all hormones are some of the most potent medicines we have in our little black bag arsenal, because they do exactly what we want them to, and we know exactly how they work. If your hormone levels are too low, the body is not able to do the functions it normally performs.

You see, hormones like steroids, like testosterone, are messengers that the brain uses to tell a cell what to do. The brain uses glands, like the testes, to send out this message. That message may be to grow, not grow, divide, not divide, go faster, go slower, and so on. Hormones really don't do anything except tell other cells what to do.

Be aware that when we talk about testosterone, there are a lot of myths, but the fact is that men with the lowest levels of testosterone have the highest causes of death, independent of age and cause. Testosterone increases muscle mass, mental function, and strength.

Does Testosterone Cause Acne?

In some cases, it's a fact; in some cases, it's a myth.

There's a component of testosterone that causes the pores and the glands on the shoulders to produce more of the product that can clog the ducts and cause acne. In men who are on high-dose testosterone, it's not uncommon that I see a rash extending from the lower part of the beard area to the upper shoulder area that's related to testosterone.

But if you're talking about facial (cystic) acne, there's very little evidence showing that testosterone is related to it. If anything is related to testosterone, it's more about the change in the level of testosterone than the testosterone itself.

Testosterone and Cancer

One of the other big misconceptions about testosterone is that it causes cancer.

As I explained, testosterone itself doesn't "do" anything. It tells the cells to grow, and it gives messages. But one of the messages it doesn't give to cells is "become cancer."

Cancer is caused when DNA inside a cell has been damaged. The DNA is the handbook that the cell uses to build all the proteins that make it do all the functions a cell does. When that handbook gets damaged, the cell doesn't work as well. And if the damage continues down the line, it eventually becomes unresponsive to the body's signals and acts on its own, doing its own thing. The cell grows without any checks and balances in place.

That's what cancer is. It's caused by damage to the DNA, which can be caused by cell division. Every time you divide a cell, you have to replicate that DNA, and there are transmission errors in the construction of the future DNA that result in the replicated DNA not being exactly like the mother cell. That damage keeps getting passed along and worsens as the cell continues to divide further and further down the line.

So that's one way of damaging the DNA. Other ways include

ultraviolet radiation, free radicals, environmental toxins, and trauma. Those all cause damage to the DNA, and from that damage, cancer can develop. Once a cancer cell develops, the testosterone may tell that cell to grow. It's not that testosterone is involved in the development of the cancer, but testosterone might cause the cancer to grow once the cancer develops.

In fact, testosterone actually causes prostate cancer cells that are abnormal to die off. That's right! Testosterone is one of the hormones that signal for prostate cells to die if that signal is not countered by another process inside the cell. That's one of the reasons that when testosterone levels are their highest, such as in eighteen to twenty-five-year-old men, we rarely see prostate cancer.

We have always heard that testosterone causes prostate cancer; that's just not true. However, testosterone may cause certain prostate cancers to grow at a faster speed.

Preventing and Alleviating Andropause Symptoms

There's much that men can do in their early years to stave off andropause.

As I've mentioned, you need to maintain an exercise habit, get proper nutrition, employ good stress management techniques, and get enough sleep. All of these methods help preserve testosterone further into your life. But eventually, no matter who you are, the cells that produce testosterone decrease or die off at a rate of 1 to 2 percent per year. Eventually, when you get old enough, your testosterone isn't going to be high enough to maintain the function that it's supposed to in the body.

Let's talk first about nutrition as it relates to andropause. It's very clear that processed foods and carbohydrates decrease a man's testosterone levels. So having a nutritional plan that's filled with good quality protein, such as chicken, as well as fresh vegetables and fruit and whole grains is the best way to avoid decreasing your testosterone level. It has to do with the endocrine system and metabolism of the body and how sugar interacts with the body to lower your testosterone level.

If your diet is filled with whole fruits and vegetables, quality protein, and good oils, you generally don't have nutrition deficiencies. Some of these nutrients that are extremely beneficial for a man in his younger years are used in the construction of testosterone.

But what's also very important is making sure that men are able to eliminate their estrogen in a healthy and timesaving manner. That is because testosterone in men is actually converted to estrogen before it is actually eliminated from the body. Estrogen itself is the hormone that tells the brain to turn off the signal that tells the testes to make more testosterone.

Nowadays, men are converting testosterone to estrogen at a high rate. The reason could be genetic, or it could be because of too much fat tissue. Fat tissue contains the enzyme aromatase, which does the conversion. Men can actually inadvertently turn down their own testosterone levels by having too much fat.

Some of the things that men need to have in their diet are what we call cruciferous vegetables. These are all the vegetables that your mom always wanted you to eat, such as broccoli, asparagus, cauliflower, cabbage, and Brussels sprouts. Eating enough of those vegetables, which contain a substance called indole-3-carbonol, helps the body metabolize the estrogen out of your system. In this manner, it can turn off the signal (estrogens) that tells your body not to produce more testosterone.

Diagnosing Andropause

To find out if he has andropause, the first thing a man needs to do is get a good doctor who can do a thorough medical history, because it's in the symptoms that you define the condition.

Because if a man has no symptoms of low testosterone, but is known to have a low normal testosterone level, it really is probably normal for him. The first thing I always tell patients is to look for the symptoms: low libido, erectile dysfunction, inability to maintain muscle mass, fatigue, and depression with anxiety. Those are the most common symptoms of low testosterone.

After a doctor diagnoses andropause, there are a number of ways in which testosterone levels can be measured. All of them have pluses and minuses. There really isn't one way that's best, but the most popular way of testing for low testosterone is through a serum blood test.

I always recommend to physicians to not test for just the total testosterone but to look for free testosterone levels. You see, since testosterone is made from cholesterol and since cholesterol is in the fat, testosterone is a fat, too. And the blood system is mostly water, and we all know that oil and water - fats and water - don't mix. The body needs to transport the testosterone through the blood system inside of the protein to keep it away from water in the body so they don't repel each other.

However, when testosterone is in this protein that we call sex hormone-binding globulin, it's not able to do the work on the cellular level that the body needs done. A man may have a "normal" level of testosterone but have a sex hormone-binding globulin that's so elevated that the amount of free testosterone actually available to do work is very low.

I think it's very important for men to seek out doctors who understand how to properly dose testosterone and the best possible way to get the effects you want without the side effects you don't want.

I'm a big advocate of not using topical testosterone gels and creams because of the odor they can give off and because of the quantity of testosterone they deliver. A normal, healthy twenty-five-year-old man produces between 8 and 12 milligrams of testosterone per day. Yet

---

some doctors prescribe gels that provide 5000 milligrams every day. That's five hundred times more testosterone than a man needs! Most of it doesn't get absorbed; their loved ones, their spouses, their kids, and their pets get exposed to it. I think these topical treatments have some real problems.

Testosterone by injection or pellet is the preferred method of treatment, once you get to the point of needing to supplement testosterone. I always tell my patients the best things to do are to stick to a good exercise and nutritional plan, manage stress, and get plenty of sleep. And, then, if your testosterone still remains low, seek out a trained physician for proper administration of testosterone to alleviate your symptoms and avoid unwanted side effects.

It is extremely important to have a physician that understands the role estrogen plays in maintaining a man's health. Testosterone is converted to estrogens, specifically estradiol. Estrogens are known for their potentially dangerous effects on the prostate as well as countering the other desirable effects of testosterone. Measuring the estradiol level is as important as measuring the free testosterone level. Maintaining a healthy but not elevated level of estradiol is imperative to a man's good health.

Finally, a man's physician will need to monitor the marker for prostate cancer called the prostate-specific antigen (PSA) and, at minimum, conduct yearly checks of a man's prostate through a manual rectal examination. Sorry guys - it goes with the territory.

Dr. Paul Savage, MD

Dr. Paul Savage is an acknowledged expert in the field of anti-aging and regenerative medicine. He is board certified by the American Academy of Anti-Aging Medicine (A4M) as well as a Fellow of Anti-Aging and Regenerative Medicine. His primary goal of regaining and maintaining optimum health for his patients as the best method of preventing disease is well established.

After training in the specialty field of Emergency Medicine and Trauma, Dr. Savage was an attending trauma physician at Grace Hospital/Detroit Receiving. His own ill health after these years of intense stress led Dr. Savage on a personal quest to improve his condition. Only a few years later, Dr. Paul Savage became one of the acknowledged experts in the field of anti-aging and was even featured in Suzanne Somers' best-selling book, *Ageless*. Dedicated and inspired to help others, Dr. Savage is the founder of a network of anti-aging centers throughout America.

Paul Savage, MD received his degree in Mathematics at Michigan State University and was educated at the University of Michigan School of Medicine – one of the premier and finest medical institutions in the country – graduating at age twenty-five. Dr. Savage has been practicing anti-aging medicine since 2002.

Information as to his current practice in Chicago can be located at www.vidabem.com.

Dr. Paul Savage
150 E Huron Street, Suite 802
Chicago IL 60611

Phone: 312-981-4020
E-mail: pesavagemd@vidabem.com
www.vidabem.com

CHAPTER NINE

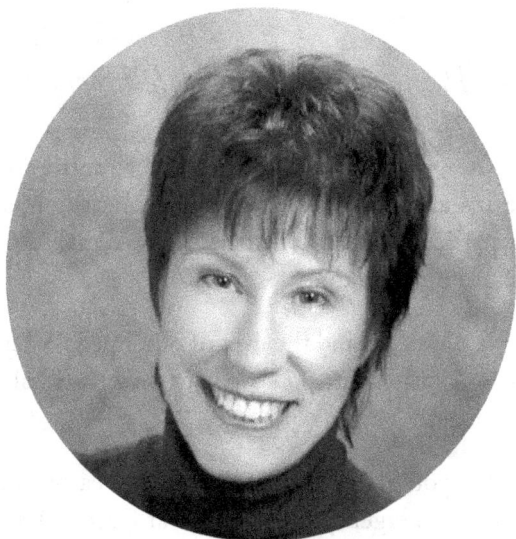

Dr. Pamela Smith:

Female Hormones

CHAPTER NINE

Dr. Pamela Smith: Female Hormones

A s a doctor, you want to look at a patient's entire body and make sure it's all in balance – hormones, nutrition, and exercise. My particular areas of expertise are female hormones and bioidentical hormone therapy.

When you are a physician and the lives of other people depend on you, it's especially important that you keep your own body balanced so you can be a good doctor.

I'm going to tell you a story about me. In my early forties, while I was working as an emergency room doctor at Detroit Medical Center, I suddenly had trouble sleeping. Nothing had changed in my work or home life. I went through eleven doctors; every single one of them told me to take a sleeping pill.

At that time, I was fortunate and happened to be attending the very first anti-aging conference. During the second seminar, the second slide mentioned that women without progesterone frequently have insomnia. No one I had talked to had mentioned the word progesterone, which is the steroid hormone that is involved in menstruation and prepares a woman's body for pregnancy. (It is lost as we age.)

When I returned home from the conference, I took a test, and the result showed that I had no progesterone. I took the bioidentical form of it, and within forty-eight hours, I was sleeping like a baby.

It was a blessing in disguise for me. By the time the next conference came around, I had left emergency medicine and had spent the last thirteen years in my new career - treating my patients by using a metabolic, anti-aging approach.

First off, let's talk about hormones. What are hormones?

Hormones are naturally produced body chemicals that send signals from cells in one part of the body to cells in another part of the body, telling them to do whatever job or task they must do. Bioidentical hormones are ones that contain the same chemical structure with which you're born. They don't necessarily have to come from plants, but in North America, they often do come from soy sources.

In women, there is a hormone called pregnenolone, which is known as the "mother hormone" and is the precursor to such hormones as estrogen, testosterone, DHEA, androgen, and eventually, progesterone.

One of the conditions women most associate with aging—and often fear — is menopause. It can begin between the ages of forty-five and fifty-five, according to the National Institutes of Health. The ovaries stop producing eggs and progesterone, less estrogen is made, and the monthly period stops.

Symptoms of menopause include hot flashes, night sweats, insomnia, decreased sexual desire, heart palpitations, mood swings, urinary leakage, forgetfulness, and vaginal dryness. Menopause is complete after a woman has not had a menstrual cycle in the past twelve months. (Men also go through a period of declining hormones that's been described as "male menopause.")

I'm a menopausal woman, and personally, I believe that menopause is the best time in a woman's life. You don't have to worry about becoming pregnant, and as long as your hormones are balanced and you can maintain all your functions, it truly is a fabulous time of life. There is no reason today that a woman should dread menopause. It's important to treat the symptoms, but this is otherwise a natural, normal process of aging.

The time when estrogen starts depleting in a woman varies for everyone. There are, in fact, three types of estrogen in women: estrone (E1), estradiol (E2), and estriol (E3). We don't want to replace E1, which is produced during menopause. E2 is the predominant form in non-pregnant women and is tied to four hundred bodily functions, including helping to lower cholesterol and blood pressure, maintain memory, and prevent cataracts. E3 is the primary estrogen of pregnancy and has been found to help prevent breast cancer.

So when we replace estrogen, we replace E2 and E3. If a woman didn't lose estrogen while she was still having her menstrual cycle, she might still be producing estrogen at sixty or seventy years old, as I've observed in some women in my practice.

More commonly, women lose progesterone first, particularly in North America. (Asian women, who have fewer menopause symptoms, have a soy-based diet and by-and-large healthier diet.) Symptoms of progesterone loss are anxiety, irritability, insomnia, depression, racing heart, bladder problems, and gut disturbances. So it's important to replace. If women have a lot of estrogen – a condition called estrogen dominance – they have an increased risk of breast cancer unless we give them progesterone to balance it out. (I go into more detail on these hormones in my book, *What You Must Know about Women's Hormones.*)

How do we go about replacing those depleted hormones? It's very important that we measure and re-measure a woman's hormone levels to find them the right balance. Studies have shown that using a blood test isn't accurate in measuring hormone levels, because it doesn't show what's going on in the body's tissues. When we give hormones externally – on the skin – it goes into the red blood cells for three seconds, then leaves. So you really can't measure it in the blood, and it has caused some people to overdose. We measure hormone levels by giving a salivary test and a twenty-four-hour urine test. Both of these give us an idea of what's going on in the entire body.

The way we give the hormones depends on the patient. We never give estrogen by mouth, as it lowers growth hormone, which helps keep us young. Taking it by mouth is also very hard on the liver and gall bladder and produces more of the E1 estrogen – the one that we don't want to be there. We usually deliver estrogen on the skin.

Some doctors use synthetic hormones such as Premarin and progestin in replacement therapies. Premarin, which is derived from the urine of pregnant mares, does contain the good E2 estrogen, but also E1; studies show we shouldn't replace it. Some confusion also comes from the use of the word progestin, which is a synthetic form of progesterone and sounds very similar. Progestin can cause anxiety, mood swings, insomnia, and depression and can cause coronary artery spasms and a higher risk of breast cancer. Progesterone helps balance out estrogen, which is not true of progestin.

Another very important body part to keep in balance is the thyroid. The thyroid, the largest adrenal gland in the body, does a lot of work to regulate every single function in the human body. So it's important to make sure it's working optimally. We want to make sure a person's thyroid-stimulating hormone, or TSH, is within an acceptable range. Some nutritional deficiencies such as iodide and the B vitamins can affect the thyroid. Conversely, too much copper and calcium can have adverse effects on the thyroid.

It's especially important for women that we get the entire picture of how the thyroid is working, because so many hormones interact with it: cortisol, progesterone, and insulin. As healthcare companies/ physicians cut costs, most doctors only measure TSH and thyroxine (T4) but not triiodothyronine (T3). They need to measure all three and see if there are also any thyroid antibodies to get a more complete picture of its health.

If your thyroid is left unregulated, your blood sugar can go up, and when that happens, insulin also rises. Insulin is the hormone that helps the body keep blood sugar in check. Pre-diabetes or full-blown diabetes can follow. Diabetes can then lead to further health concerns, such as high blood pressure, cancer, and memory loss.

You can try to stave off diabetes by eating a low-glycemic index diet of "good carbs" – those foods that generally have less of an impact on blood sugar levels. These foods include fruits, vegetables, legumes, and whole and minimally processed grains. Exercise and fiber often help as well, as can chromium and some herbs. There are nutrients such as cinnamon that can be added to your food to reduce blood sugar.

In my opinion, the most important thing is to eat breakfast. When you don't eat breakfast, you set your body up for influences from toxins. I believe you should eat breakfast before 10 a.m. to be healthy and certainly within an hour of waking up, even if you aren't hungry. If you're the kind of person who's not hungry when you wake up, then we already know your insulin isn't working as effectively as it could.

Another important thing to include in a health-centered diet is Omega fatty acids, especially Omega 3, which is found in fish oil and is an ant-inflammatory. You can also use Omega 9, which is in olive oil. Omega 3, when a mother takes it during pregnancy, has been shown to increase IQ and reduce ADD and dyslexia in her children. There are so many nutrients that are important, but if you only take one, Omega 3 should be it.

Men and women everywhere want to stay healthy. Many of us will live to be a hundred years old, but no one wants to live to be a hundred if they go into a nursing home at age eighty. Metabolic anti-aging medicine is all about staying healthy and maintaining vision, memory, and mobility. To do this, you need to be hormonally balanced. And now that we've developed such wonderful anti-aging and bioidentical hormone replacement therapies, it's much easier to live a long, healthy life.

Dr. Pamela Smith

Dr. Pamela Wartian Smith is an internationally known speaker and best-selling author in the fields of anti-aging and functional and metabolic medicine.

After earning her medical degree at Meharry Medical College in 1978, Dr. Smith spent her first twenty years of practice as an emergency room physician with the Detroit Medical Center. She went on to earn a master's degree in public health from the Medical College of Wisconsin. She's also a Diplomate of the Board of the American Academy of Anti-Aging Physicians.

Dr. Smith is the founder and director of the Center for Healthy Living and Longevity with offices in Michigan and Florida. She is also the founder and director of The Fellowship in Metabolic, Anti-Aging and Functional Medicine and the Co-director of the master's program in Medical Sciences with a concentration in Metabolic and Nutritional Medicine at the University of South Florida College of Medicine.

Dr. Smith has been featured on CNN, PBS, and other television stations. She has been interviewed in numerous consumer magazines and has hosted two of her own radio shows. She's the author of the best-selling books, *HRT: The Answers, Vitamins: Hype or Hope, Demystifying Weight Loss, What You Must Know about Vitamins, Minerals, Herbs & More, and What You Must Know about Women's Hormones.* Her newest book, *Why You Can't Lose Weight*, is scheduled to be released shortly.

Dr. Pamela Smith
Traverse City Office
Suite G02, 13919 S West Bay Shore Drive
Traverse City, Michigan, United States
49684

Phone: 231-929-7450
E-mail: faafm63@yahoo.com
www.cfhll.com

CHAPTER TEN

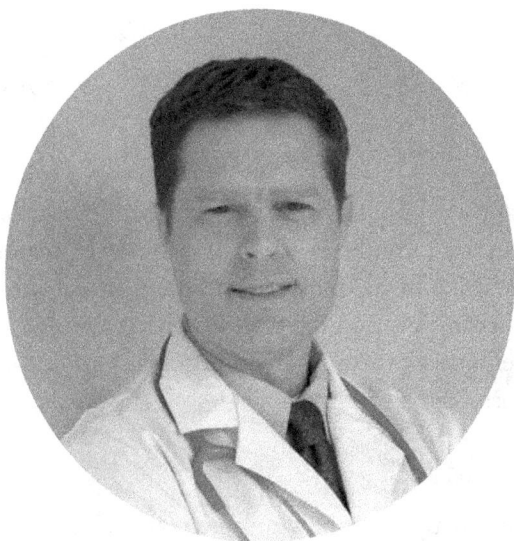

Dr. Screven Edgerton:

Perimenopause

CHAPTER TEN

Dr. Screven Edgerton: Perimenopause

A woman goes through many changes over her life span: from infant to child, from adolescent to fully developed woman, often into motherhood, and ultimately maturing into a senior citizen. One of the most pivotal times in her life is the onset of her menstrual cycle and, later in life, its cessation. From regular cycles to menopause, there is a subtle transition that occurs called perimenopause.

Defining Perimenopause

Perimenopause is the time between premenopause (regular cycles of ovulation) and menopause (permanent infertility). Premenopause is when the ovaries are functioning perfectly and there's perfect harmony among all of the body's hormones. Menopause is the time where many of the major hormones are in decline or at a deficiency state.

It's during perimenopause that a woman's body undergoes biologic changes as her ovaries begin to produce less of the female sex hormones. In this middle zone, there are good levels of some hormones and others that are starting to fall. It's the imbalance of hormones that can cause many of a woman's unpleasant symptoms.

Women begin this transition at different ages: some prematurely as early as their thirties but most others in their forties. Perimenopause can last more than six years, though four years is the average. A woman is considered to have reached full menopause after she has gone 12 consecutive months without a menstrual period.

The symptoms of perimenopause, which can be wide-ranging, can include the following:

- Irregular (longer, shorter, heavier, or lighter) periods
- Menstrual cycles that are more or less than twenty-eight days apart
- Hot flashes or hot flushes
- Mood changes/mood swings
- Sleep problems/insomnia
- Vaginal dryness
- "Foggy" brain or lack of mental clarity

Many of these symptoms mimic what you would experience during menopause. I think it's important to address your individual symptoms with your physician. I believe many practitioners fall short by treating women as if they were in complete menopause. It really doesn't have to be as aggressive as that.

As a patient of mine goes through this change, I try to put her best interests first and help her cope with her symptoms in the most scientific way possible. I also look at natural options such as bioidentical hormones (hormones that are the same as what your body produces) for treatment. Balancing mainstream medicine and natural treatments has served me – and my patients - well throughout my career.

It's about finding out which hormones may be deficient, replacing them, and monitoring the patient's hormone levels. As a doctor, you need to make sure the hormones that don't need replacing continue to be produced at normal levels. If you restore balance in the perimenopausal woman, then you've empowered her body to coast very naturally and happily into menopause.

I have found that progesterone is the first hormone to get sluggish in the perimenopausal phase of a woman's life. Typically, a woman's ovaries continue to produce an adequate amount of estrogen. Because of the aging process, either the number of ovulations declines or the quality of egg production is diminished. This translates into less production of progesterone (the pro-gestational hormone).

There is a delicate balance between estrogen and progesterone. So when progesterone starts to become under produced and estrogen continues to be produced normally, then there's a mismatch. A lot of people use the term estrogen-dominant, which I'm not particularly fond of as a clinical term, because that implies that somebody is making too much estrogen. I think the more correct term would be progesterone-deficient.

Much of the time, treatment is as easy as giving a woman bioidentical progesterone to recreate that healthy balance between estrogen and progesterone. We then see the symptoms that mimic menopause really start to fade away, and a woman's body behaves in a regular fashion without a hormone deficiency.

Your doctor will have to re-evaluate your hormone levels as you get a little older. If he starts to see other hormones decline, then s/he can re-address hormone treatment and help you coast into menopause without suffering through the usual symptoms.

The Importance of Diet and Nutrition

A healthy diet can play an important role in helping a woman age gracefully.

Everyone should have a balanced diet. If a woman can limit the amount of processed food that she eats, then her body is going to react better overall. The body won't be stripped of minerals, and energy levels will continue to be maintained properly. The focus should be on eating fresh, whole fruits and vegetables close to their source of origin and limiting the consumption of processed, fast, and fried foods. Many of the properties of fresh, non-processed foods actually assist the body with hormone metabolism. Often, the processing of hormones can follow a harmful metabolism pathway that is a set up for disease states and possibly cancer.

By eating "cleaner," your body is going to be more empowered to have a healthy gastrointestinal tract, which can absorb nutrients, supplements, and hormones better. A lot of good health comes back to your GI tract, so diet is crucial to keeping the GI tract healthy. Seventy percent of our immunity lives within the gastrointestinal tract. Additionally, many of the amino acids used in our brain are produced in the gut. For example, much of the serotonin in our brain is made from the GI tract. Serotonin is a neurotransmitter that regulates many bodily functions, including mood, appetite, and sensory perception. Ultimately, if the GI tract is optimized, then food, supplements, medications, and so on can all be absorbed more efficiently. Immunity and hormone regulation is optimal when the gastrointestinal tract is at its best.

Diet and vitamins are crucial to healthy living, especially during times of hormone fluctuation. In addition to a healthy diet, a woman should take a high-quality multivitamin with a full B vitamin complement. This B vitamin will allow a woman's body to thrive in the face of hormone deficiency as her doctor is replacing the hormones that are deficient during perimenopause. Other important supplements are Omega fish oils and Vitamin D. These are the three standard things I recommend.

Growing Awareness of Perimenopause

I think that in recent years, the medical community and the public are getting better about understanding the transition a woman's body makes from being premenopausal to completely menopausal. Furthermore, we are realizing this change doesn't happen overnight. That change is not a switch that just gets flipped; it's a transition. The change facing a woman is going from hormone equilibrium to hormone deficiency.

Our understanding now is that the shift from premenopause to menopause does not happen all at once. This fact allows doctors to replenish the hormone deficiencies that are happening in real time. By doing this, we avoid over-treating patients. Unfortunately, many doctors still tell women that their collection of symptoms sounds like menopause. They then give the patient a whole complement of menopausal treatment, often resulting in more side effects than benefits. Women then go off their treatment regimen and are then back to square one, leaving them more miserable than they were in the first place.

So I think it's important for doctors to pay attention to the details and the subtleties of how a woman transitions from pure premenopause to pure menopause. This allows us to treat our patients, make them happier, and avoid a lot of uncomfortable and unnecessary symptoms.

By treating women with hormone deficiency early, we are getting a jump on preventative health. Hormone replacement promotes cardiac, colon, bone, and brain health. When women do not replace their deficient hormones, we inevitably see higher rates of cardiovascular disease, bone disease, and poorer overall mortality. Treating the symptoms of hormone deficiency makes the patient feel better but truly is secondary to the overall health benefits that are ultimately garnered from natural hormone replacement.

By treating patients appropriately, without over-treatment in the perimenopausal phase, we have provided them a true health service in addition to addressing the symptoms for which they came to us in the first place.

Dr. Screven Edgerton

Dr. Screven T. Edgerton is a board-certified obstetrician and gynecologist and the co-owner of Balanced Hormones and Health in Austin, Texas.

He has an interest and very specialized training in bioidentical hormone replacement and in preventative medicine and treatment.

Balanced Hormones and Health was born of a unique collaboration between doctor and patient. Registered nurse Tracy Ganske was thirty-two years old when doctors misdiagnosed a case of severe hypothyroidism, which is easily controlled with a simple hormone treatment. After successful treatment, she became a partner with Dr. Edgerton in this new practice.

Their goal is to focus on diet, nutrition, pharmaceutical-grade supplements, sophisticated diagnostic testing, and bioidentical hormone replacement as an alternative to mainstream prescription medications. This natural approach optimizes energy, fitness and overall well-being.

Dr. Edgerton is a native of Louisiana, who graduated from Vanderbilt University with an undergraduate degree in biology in 1995. He earned his Doctor of Medicine from Louisiana State University. He completed his training in obstetrics and gynecology and was chief resident at The University of Texas in Houston in 2005.

He is a member of the American Medical Association and Texas Association of Obstetricians and Gynecologists and a Fellow of the American College of Obstetrics & Gynecology.

Dr. Screven Edgerton
1010 West 9th Street
Austin, Texas, United States
78703

Phone: 512-410-2518
E-mail: info@balancedhormonesandhealth.com
www.balancedhormonesandhealth.com

CHAPTER ELEVEN

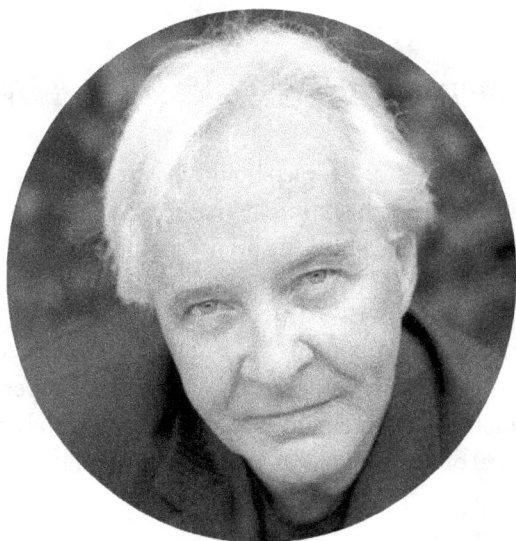

Dr. Andrew Wojcicki:

Human Growth Hormone

CHAPTER ELEVEN

Dr. Andrew Wojcicki: Human Growth Hormone

My life's motto: People should live in harmony with nature. I believe it's the only way that we can maintain the balance of our body's physical and psychological needs for long life and health.

Harmonizing these components of your body – diet, activity level, and mental well-being — is necessary as you age. Proper energy and nutrients, which create an environment where your body can produce the desired level of healthy cells, is known as preventative or anti-aging medicine.

The bottom line is that science shows us that 80 percent of the diseases associated with aging – including cancer – are preventable. But the prevention of these types of diseases depends on our lifestyle.

Any interference of external factors such as doctors and medications should be a last resort for your treatment. I believe that complementary treatments – not replacements, and nothing to the extreme – will improve your body's natural processes.

Apart from external influences and lifestyle, the effects of hormones on your body are critical. They can answer the questions: How long are you going to live? How are you going to live? How healthy will that life be? There certainly is an expected and predicted range of human life expectancy, but within this spectrum, exactly how long and how healthy that life is depends very much on us.

The discovery of the human growth hormone and its functions is a fairly recent one – within the last sixty or seventy years. It's abundant in the human body during puberty, the time when we are growing faster and undergoing our "growth spurts."

We've learned that human growth hormone is necessary not just during this early period, but throughout our whole lives. The growth hormone continues to produce throughout adult life and remains the most abundant hormone in the adult pituitary gland. Also, all body tissues examined today contain receptors for GH.

Hormones are named after the Greek God Hermes (the messenger), because hormones send messages to the body, telling it what to do and how to do it. In any part of our body, be it the heart or brain, there is always a factor that's ready to receive stimulation, or a message, from its growth hormone to continue functioning.

The first signs of aging start to occur between the ages of twenty-five and thirty when you start to experience a decline in the growth hormone. And, again, growth hormone is pivotal.

It is, in fact, a regenerative hormone, so that even if a person's tissue is to some degree deteriorated or damaged, it can still be regenerated by the growth hormone. To what extent the growth hormone can regenerate tissue is not yet fully known, but, fortunately, more and more scientists are getting interested in this hormone, which is a very essential part of us.

Studies in Sweden, Denmark, and Australia show that there is tremendous benefit to taking growth hormone. Very minor side effects – which happen very rarely and can be corrected by adjusting the dose – are carpal tunnel syndrome and fluid retention. Some of the conditions that can be prevented or managed by the growth hormone include osteoporosis and heart disease.

Several studies have shown that a deficiency of the human growth hormone is linked to the slowing down of the pituitary gland, called hypopituitarism, and has a negative effect on life expectancy.

Therefore, preventing growth hormone deficiency syndrome has a very significant impact on a person's quality of life. When you're lacking growth hormone, your body's aging mechanisms will accelerate, and you'll experience an increase in body fat, reduced muscle bulk, decreased strength and physical fitness, less sweating, impaired psychological well-being, depression, and increased anxiety risk.

Hypopituitarism can lead to obesity and cardiovascular disease such as cardiomyopathy. Cardiomyopathy is the weakening of the muscles of the heart and the failure of the heart to pump. I'm convinced that, in addition to its many anti-aging applications, growth hormone should be used for cardiomyopathy patients.

There is another area where growth hormone can be used – surgery. It's particularly helpful in treating orthopedic conditions like hip or knee replacement and in open-heart surgery. Healing is shown to improve with the use of growth hormone – both before and after surgery, reducing hospitalization and speeding up recovery.

The growth hormone gene involved in healing damaged tissue was discovered and described by Dr. Robert Costa, a professor of biochemistry and molecular genetics at the University of Illinois in Chicago. It can help explain why we age. His focus has been on the FoxM1B gene, which is a part of the entire life cycle of the cells of all mammals. This gene helps control cell division, and its activity is elevated in younger mammals and diminished in older ones. When the gene's effects are diminished, cells can't regenerate in a normal way, and this can lead to loss of elasticity, muscle atrophy, and slower healing of wounds. More recent studies show that using growth hormone therapy has a positive effect on the gene, allowing cells to grow the way they did in younger mammals.

Growth hormone can also be very helpful in treating osteoporosis, which is a condition that's characterized by low bone mass, a deterioration of bone tissue, leading to fragile bones and a higher risk of fractures, according to the National Osteoporosis Foundation. In a 1996 study in the Annals of Internal Medicine, growth hormone therapy was shown to increase bone density and make it healthier in comparison to other treatments. One year of growth hormone therapy led to a significant improvement in bone density and in treating osteoporosis. This effect lasted five to ten years after the treatment was stopped.

Studies have also shown that those people who were treated with growth hormone were more inclined to exercise and took less sick leave – three times less, according to a 2001 study – *(Clinical Endocrinal Metabolism 86:5277-52814, 2001 E. Hernberg-Stahl)* than their counterparts with growth hormone deficiency. Those deficient also had hospital stays that were twice as long and required 30 percent more assistance with daily activities over their peers who had good hormone levels.

There are natural ways to increase the body's level of growth hormone. The first way is exercise. Moderate cardiovascular, aerobic exercise is the most effective and is recommended. Spending hours in the gym will actually lower the level of growth hormone and deplete Q10, which is present in cells and helps produce most of the body's energy. For people over fifty, exercise shouldn't be more than three times a week for forty-five minutes. Of those forty-five minutes, thirty minutes should be for cardiovascular exercise and the other fifteen dedicated to muscle-toning work. This regimen will best stimulate growth hormone.

Food is also very important in creating growth hormone. You should consume non-contaminated proteins and meats. By non-contaminated, I mean unaffected by added steroids. I recommend people stick to organic/hormone-free sources of proteins. Carbohydrates reduce the level of growth hormone, so avoiding them in your diet – especially refined, processed carbs – is key.

As far as the human growth hormone oral supplements or powder you see in health food stores, there's something you ought to know: Often, what's most likely included in the powder is L-Arginine. L-Arginine is an amino acid that stimulates your pituitary gland to increase its level of growth hormone. I do not recommend this treatment, as what is commonly seen is a wide variety of additives combined with L-Arginine that are unnecessary and may contain steroids. Additionally, if a problem exists with an unresponsive pituitary gland, there will be a reduced effect. The real human growth hormone replacement treatment is done by subcutaneous injections, followed by a medical doctor monitoring benefits or adverse yet reversible side effects. How do you know if you are deficient? One test that's used to see if people qualify to take human growth hormone is to stimulate their pituitary gland and see if it is functioning enough. If it's not, then you can add the growth hormone. Blood work is also a common way to determine levels of GH present in your system.

Over the years, there's been a stigma attached to the words "human growth hormone." Why is this? Very often, growth hormone has been used and abused. Sports professionals studying and using growth hormone saw that energy and cellular metabolism levels increased.

So they started using it just for the purpose of achieving short-term goals: winning medals, breaking a record, or making money, instead of for living a long and healthy life. People often mistake growth hormone with steroids, which it is not. I think this is why people have a negative association with growth hormone.

Many people take thyroid hormone or insulin, and nobody considers this extreme. Why then should GH be treated any differently? Millions of people need to take them to be alive and well. I don't consider that to be "playing God" (as some might believe) when we add hormones to our bodies. Like anything else, hormones are extremely useful when used judiciously.

We have a basic idea of what level of growth hormone is good, but it's a very individual thing. Any time I treat a patient with growth hormone, it has to be based on his/her specific needs. Some may need more hormones, some less; some sooner in life, some later. These "bioidentical" hormones I use are plant-based hormones that are made to be identical to the ones our body produces and to not cause harm. Our body recognizes them as being part of its natural make-up and accepts them.

If we look back one hundred years, human life expectancy was about fifty years. Now, as science and medical treatments have improved, our life expectancy is seventy or eighty years in the developed world. That's progress!

The number one thing people want in life is to feel good and feel healthy. I believe that by employing growth hormone therapy, you can keep your body in balance and healthy for a long time.

Dr. Andrew Wojcicki

A native of Poland and an orthopedic surgeon before his immigration to Canada, Dr. Andrew Wojcicki is a well-known and respected gerontologist and internal medicine specialist.

After studying at the University of Toronto upon his arrival in Canada, Dr. Wojcicki dedicated his career to the prevention of aging-related diseases. He is well known for innovative therapies that help to prevent specific conditions related to hormonal changes and the effects of aging.

Now, as the medical director of Vivian Medical Spa (alongside his wife Anna, a radiation oncologist) in Mount Albert, Ontario, Dr. Wojcicki treats his patients with balancing hormones first, lifestyle assessments, nutrition supplements, intravenous treatments for cardiovascular support and cancer prevention, and body detoxification treatments including balneotherapy, a branch of medicine that concentrates on the therapeutic value of baths, especially those taken with natural mineral waters (in this case, Austrian moor mud bath therapies).

Dr. Wojcicki is a fellow of the Royal College of Physicians and Surgeons of Canada and a fellow of the American Academy of Anti-Aging Medicine. He also works at Southlake Regional Health Centre in Newmarket, Ontario, as staff Internist and Gerontologist.

Dr. Andrew Wojcicki
Vivian Medical Spa
6165 Vivian Road
Mount Albert, Ontario, Canada
L0G 1M0

Phone: 905-473-1435
E-mail: info@vivianmedicalspa.com
www.vivianmedicalspa.com

AFTERWORD

This book is only the beginning. We hope that we have helped you to identify, prevent, and care for some of the conditions associated with aging and empowered you to stay proactive about your health and wellness. As doctors, all of us take what we do very seriously and have spent many extra hours training in this field so that we can give you the best and most up-to-date treatments possible.

In the above chapters, we've touched upon hormone-related conditions and therapies; diabetes and its related diseases; perimenopause and menopause; testosterone loss and andropause; detoxification; inflammation; pellet therapy; adrenal fatigue; and the manner in which your dental health reflects your overall health.

It's inevitable that we age, but now it's possible to age in a way that's very different from that of our parents and grandparents. If you look back a hundred years, human life expectancy was about fifty years. Today, our life expectancy is seventy or eighty years in the developed world.

Improved technology and more widespread acknowledgment and acceptance of hormone replacement with bioidentical hormones has made it possible for you to live out your golden years as an active, well-balanced, healthy, and happy human being. Our goal as anti-aging specialists is to get all of your hormones in harmony so you can be the best, healthiest you – the version of you that nature intended.

Much of what we've discussed boils down to the concepts of living an active lifestyle; eating whole, fresh, natural foods; reducing highly processed carbohydrates and sugars; getting regular visits with your doctor to discuss what's going on with your body; and getting your hormone levels checked.

Once we get your hormones to their natural levels by correcting any deficits, your body will respond as if it's a person much younger. You'll feel better - much more like your "old self."

Also, many health conditions we see today are exacerbated by the prevalence of environmental toxins in our world. It's therefore important that you eat foods high in antioxidants and do detoxification on occasion to purge these toxins from your body and keep your system from being slowed down. Drinking lots of water also plays a key role in this process.

Another pivotal part of maintaining good health into your senior years is exercise. If you regularly participate in a physical activity that you love, you will boost your "feel good hormones" and serotonin in addition to the "runner's high" that's created by increased endorphins. You will gain muscle, strength, and bone density.

Exercise will protect you against heart disease, colds, dementia, hot flashes, gum disease, diabetes, excess body fat, and depression. It supports your immune system; improves sleep; protects your bones, joints, and vision; and improves wound healing, sex, and job performance. This adds up to less overall stress and healthier recovery from the stress we all encounter daily.

It is also critical to your overall health that you find ways to manage stress and keep the mind-body connection in balance. Breathing exercises, yoga, bubble baths, and massages all help the body relax. Getting enough sleep falls into this category, too. It doesn't matter whether the stress in your life is emotional, nutritional, or environmental: It all affects your longevity and quality of life in a negative way.

A successful anti-aging program will allow you to realize your optimal health, vitality, and longevity. If you take our advice and make a conscious choice to take good care of yourself, your long life will be a healthy one, and you will enjoy it to its fullest.

And that's what everyone wants.

To get in touch with any of the doctors featured in this book, check out www.TBookSeries.com and www.ilovemyhormonestv.com.

RECOMMENDED
RESOURCES

GET
PUBLISHED!

FREE BONUS

The Ultimate Publishing House's Production & Publicity System is so Precise, we can have your book ready in 5.5 months:

- Provides you with a professional ghostwriter
- Takes care of the hundreds of details involved in producing a book, from ISBN numbers, to marketing material to online distribution.
- Teaches you how to use your book to boost your business, get speaking engagements and media attention.
- The Top publicists and marketing experts work with us on our unique turnkey system which includes cover and book design, media kits and your own personalized website to build your personal brand.
- You have your very own personal project manager, who takes care ofall the details, while you take care of your business and he or she is accessible 24 hours a day.

**Call today to start your book,
it is the best marketing investment you will ever make!**

647 883 1758 OR EMAIL Felicia@feliciapizzonia.com

www.ultimatepublishinghouse.com

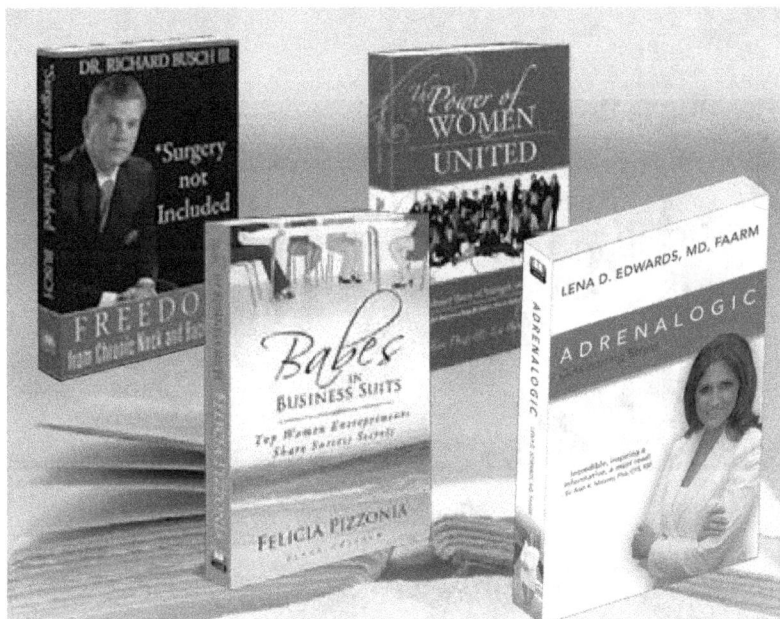

The publishing world has changed dramatically. In the new economy with global opportunities, you are either distinct or extinct, the choice is yours.

A book is the ultimate branding tool that offers:

- Credibility
- Visibility
- Distinction
- Positions you as the Expert in your field
- Media Exposure
- Attract more clients or patients
- Opportunities for product endorsements
- Its time you publish your own book with the Ultimate Publishing House!

Call today to start your book, it is the best marketing investment you will ever make!
647 883 1758 OR
EMAIL Felicia@feliciapizzonia.com

TUBA

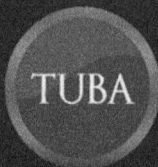

THE ULTIMATE
BRANDING AGENCY

THE ULTIMATE BRANDING AGENCY (TUBA) PINPOINTS DOCTORS AND HEALTH PROFESSIONAL TARGET MARKET BY DESIGNING A BEAUTIFUL AND FUNCTIONAL WEBSITE THAT SEAMLESSLY WORKS WITH PRECISE INTERNET MARKETING TOOLS-SOCIAL MEDIA, NAMELY; TWITTER, LINKEDIN AND YOUTUBE.

RESEARCH INDICATES THAT 80% OF ADULTS (95 MILLION AMERICANS) LOOK ONLINE FOR HEALTH AND MEDICAL INFORMATION.

AND 29% OF INTERNET USERS SEARCH ONLINE FOR A PARTICULAR DOCTOR OR MEDICAL CENTER.

HOW WELL DOES YOUR WEBSITE ATTRACT AND SERVICE THIS AUDIENCE?

DOES YOUR WEBSITE PRESENT THE PROFESSIONAL IMAGE YOU WANT TO PROJECT FOR YOUR HEALTHCARE PRACTICE?

TUBA SPECIALIZES IN THE HEALTHCARE/MEDICAL INDUSTRY AND PROVIDE COMPLETE WEBSITE DESIGN, DEVELOPMENT AND SOCIAL MEDIA IMPLEMENTATION AND MAINTENANCE. WE UNDERSTAND THE UNIQUE NEEDS OF A MEDICAL PRACTICE AND WILL...

- OVER HAUL YOUR SITE TO BE MORE RELEVANT
- DEVELOP A COMPLETE SOLUTION FROM SCRATCH
- DEVELOP A NEW LOGO AND BRANDING

THE RETURN ON INVESTMENT IS OUTSTANDING! HOW WOULD YOU FEEL IF YOU AND YOUR PRACTICE WERE ACTUALLY RANKED ON GOOGLE AND OTHER SEARCH ENGINES? THINK ABOUT THIS, LET'S SAY A POTENTIAL PATIENT CANNOT SEARCH OR FIND YOU ON GOOGLE THEN WHAT'S THE POINT OF HAVING A WEBSITE?

CALL US TODAY, WE ARE HAPPY TO HELP! PHONE 647-883-1758
OR E-MAIL US AT INFO@MEDIMARKETINGARM.COM

BOOK ORDER FORM

A D R E N A L O G I C
Outsmarting Stress

Personal Information

NAME

ADDRESS

CITY   **SUITE/APT #**

PROV/STATE   **COUNTRY**   **POSTAL/ZIP CODE**

TELEPHONE NUMBER   **FAX NUMBER**

EMAIL

$29.97   ORDER YOUR COPY TODAY!
SHIPPING $6.95

Shipping Information

PLEASE SEND PAYMENT & ORDER TO:

Ultimate Publishing House
The Ultimate Publishing House
PO Box 49540 - 80 Glen Shields Avenue
Concord, Ontario, Canada L4K 2B0

Telephone: 647-883-1758

THANK YOU FOR YOUR ORDER!

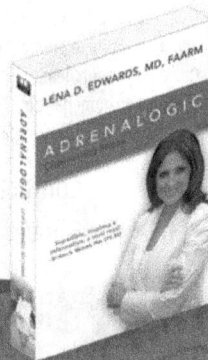

AGED *to* PERFECTION

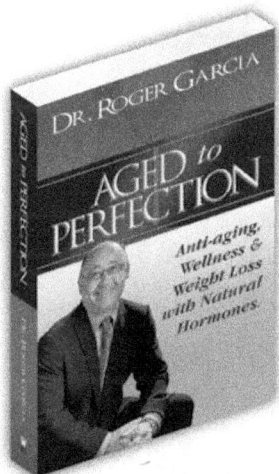

www.ingramcontent.com/pod-product-compliance
Lightning Source LLC
Chambersburg PA
CBHW050532270326
41926CB00015B/3182